Managing Stress: Before It Manages You

Managing Stress

BEFORE IT MANAGES YOU

Jenny Steinmetz
Jon Blankenship
Linda Brown
Deborah Hall
Grace Miller

BULL PUBLISHING COMPANY

P.O. Box 208, Palo Alto, Calif. 94302

ISBN Number: 0-915950-44-8

Library of Congress
Catalog Card No. 80-66389

Printed in the United States of America

Both the masculine and feminine genders will be used in this book. There was no overall plan for when we used "he" or when we used "she."

This book is dedicated to the many participants of our program, whose enthusiastic feedback and careful suggestions helped us enormously. We are most grateful to our two conscientious typists: Barbara Cannon and Debbie Heller.

Table of Contents

I

Stress— What Is It— What To Do About It?

"STRESS" IS A TERM being used more and more commonly by people to describe what ails them most in modern society. In a medical sense, stress has been described as the rate of "wear and tear within the body." There are varying degrees and different forms of stress — mental, emotional, and physical — all having an effect, sometimes positive, sometimes negative, upon health.

Stress, in fact, is an integral element of life. We are all equipped with innate "stress alarms" that allow us to react effectively in many situations. Without any stress, there would be little constructive activity. Normal excitement and pleasurable emotions may involve stress and tension, and are exhilarating. This type of stress is important and healthy, provided it is followed by a "relaxation rebound." That is, after being "wound up," the body returns to a normal level of functioning and does not carry tension beyond the time it is necesary.

Imagine the last time you felt the following symptoms:

mind going a mile a minute
body tense
hands clammy
heart beating rapidly
stomach churning

What emotions were you experiencing? Anxiety? Anger? Frustration? These are the ones most commonly reported. But do you remember the last time you were really feeling romantic, excited about someone or something, or intellectually challenged? You probably experienced many of the same physical symptoms.

Your body experiences stress when you are upset *and* when you are excited. We label the first set of emotions as negative and the second set as positive. The purpose of this stress management program is to help you reduce the amount of negative stress you experience, so that you can fully enjoy and appreciate those positive stress experiences.

The problem in our post-industrial culture today is that the degree of stress has become excessive and harmful. A rapidly-paced society—fast food, fast travel, fast fun—creates many pressures for each of us. We are constantly faced with a sense of urgency, the pressure to accomplish more and more in less and less time. Technological innovations move information and communication faster every day. Environmental and job stressors—air and noise pollution, overcrowding in the city, job deadline pressures and work overload — are increasingly present in our everyday lives. Unfortunately, many of the behaviors admired in this society contribute to a high level of stress, such as ambition, drive, extreme goal orientation, financial success and competitive spirit. This only adds to the effect of the stressors already inherent in the physical environment.

One result of this state of affairs has been the emergence of the "Type A Behavior Pattern" (Friedman and Rosenman, 1974). Type A behavior includes the presence of several or all of the following characteristics:

1. Moving, eating or walking rapidly;
2. Hurrying the ends of sentences;
3. Feeling impatient with the rate at which most things take place;
4. "Polyphasic" thought or performance (doing or thinking about 2-3 things at the same time, i.e., driving to work while shaving and/or eating breakfast);
5. Feeling guilty about relaxing or doing "nothing";
6. Thinking about business or work while on vacation;
7. Scheduling more and more in less and less time;
8. Having difficulty listening to others because of preoccupation with one's own thoughts;
9. Spending so much time acquiring things that there is no time left to enjoy them;
10. Believing that success is due to the ability to get things done quickly, and thus being afraid to stop doing everything faster and faster.

In general, "Type A" people will be aggressive and extroverted. They will have very strong personalities and may tend to dominate conversations. They have an excessive competitive drive, and a continual sense of time urgency, and may be easily aroused to anger. They are often ambitious, fiercely impatient and drive-oriented. (Pelletier, 1976).

Stress can be caused by other people. (Is there an aggressive screamer in your life?) — and by you all by yourself ("I will never learn this material!"). It is important to determine the sources of your stress as well as your common stress symptoms. Then you can try the suggestions we present in this program and determine which work the best for you in reducing or at least managing the stress in your life.

There is no way short of total isolation to eliminate the stress in our lives and, indeed, who would want to do away with joy and excitement? You will still have to deal with crazy drivers who will send your alarm system screaming. The trick is to be able to become calm quickly and to avoid prolonged stress. It is the chronic, ongoing stress (experienced at home, school, work and even competitive play) that is injurious.

In order to reduce this stress you will want to shift gears periodically throughout the day. You will want to differentiate between situations you can change and those you cannot. You will want to change some of the ways you talk to yourself.

This book is designed to give you first a sense of awareness of what causes you stress (we'll call these things *stressors*), and then to have you recognize your physical, emotional and behavioral symptoms of stress. Following this section, a number of techniques will be presented for changing your reactions to stressors, together with a number of exercises and examples to help you personalize and develop your best strategies for managing stress.

Treat this book as a clothing store. Try everything on; that way you will know what fits you. Some techniques may fit you perfectly. Others may need a tuck or two to make them right for you, and still others may not fit you at all, at least at this time. The important thing is for you to have some ways that make you feel more in control of the stress in your life: more joy and less frustration.

Exercise I-1

Take the conflict/stress questionnaire. You will notice that it is divided into three major sections. The first section asks you to look at your stress symptoms. Each of us expresses stress in a unique way. The symptoms we have listed are those which have been reported most frequently in the groups with which we have worked. The second section lists the most common forms of stress reduction. Again, we each have our own ways of relaxing. The third section lists many common stressors. Some are related to work situations, others to different types of people and still others to ways you talk to yourself. Some, but not all, should be stressful for you. There are spaces at the bottom to list other stressors in your life. Follow the instructions in each section carefully. We will use the results in the next section.

CONFLICT/STRESS QUESTIONNAIRE

I. STRESS SYMPTOMS

Which of these stress symptoms do you experience? Circle the appropriate number. The column after the "5" indicates whether it represents P (physiological stress), E (emotional stress), or B (behavioral stress).

	NEVER	RARELY	SOMETIMES	OFTEN	ALWAYS	
Headaches	1	2	3	4	5	(P)
Stomach aches or tension	1	2	3	4	5	(P)
Backaches	1	2	3	4	5	(P)
Stiffness in the neck and shoulders	1	2	3	4	5	(P)
Elevated blood pressure	1	2	3	4	5	(P)
Fatigue	1	2	3	4	5	(P)
Crying	1	2	3	4	5	(B)
Forgetfulness	1	2	3	4	5	(B)
Yelling	1	2	3	4	5	(B)
Blaming	1	2	3	4	5	(B)
Bossiness	1	2	3	4	5	(B)
Compulsive gum chewing	1	2	3	4	5	(B)

	NEVER	RARELY	SOMETIMES	OFTEN	ALWAYS	
Compulsive eating	1	2	3	4	5	(B)
Worrying	1	2	3	4	5	(E)
Depression	1	2	3	4	5	(E)
Agitation	1	2	3	4	5	(B)
Impatience	1	2	3	4	5	(E)
Anger	1	2	3	4	5	(B)
Frustration	1	2	3	4	5	(E)
Loneliness	1	2	3	4	5	(E)
Powerlessness	1	2	3	4	5	(E)
Inflexibility	1	2	3	4	5	(E)
Compulsive smoking	1	2	3	4	5	(B)
Teeth grinding	1	2	3	4	5	(B)
Other ______________	1	2	3	4	5	

II. STRESS REDUCTION

How often do you use these measures to relax?

	NEVER	RARELY	SOMETIMES	OFTEN	ALWAYS
Take aspirin	1	2	3	4	5
Use tranquilizers or other medication	1	2	3	4	5
Drink coffee, Coke, or eat frequently	1	2	3	4	5

	NEVER	RARELY	SOMETIMES	OFTEN	ALWAYS
Use relaxation techniques (meditation, yoga)	1	2	3	4	5
Use informal relaxation techniques (e.g., take time out for deep breathing, imagining pleasant scenes)	1	2	3	4	5

	NEVER	RARELY	SOMETIMES	OFTEN	ALWAYS
Exercise	1	2	3	4	5
Talk to someone you know	1	2	3	4	5
Leave your work area and go somewhere (time out, sick days, lunch away from your organization, etc.)	1	2	3	4	5
Smoke	1	2	3	4	5
Use humor	1	2	3	4	5
Have an alcoholic drink	1	2	3	4	5
Other ________________	1	2	3	4	5

III. STRESSFUL CONDITIONS

There are frequently day to day conditions which we find stressful. Go through them, reading each one, and put a check next to those that apply to you. Then go back over the checked items and indicate how often each source is true for you by circling the appropriate number.

The symbols in parentheses indicate the type of stressors: *P* (physical), *S* (social), *O* (organizational), and *ST* (self-talk).

	NEVER	RARELY	SOMETIMES	OFTEN	ALWAYS
____ 1. I am uncomfortable meeting strangers (S)/(ST)	1	2	3	4	5
____ 2. I am uncomfortable speaking in front of a group (ST)	1	2	3	4	5
____ 3. I am concerned over my ability to do everything I want to (ST)	1	2	3	4	5
____ 4. Others I work with seem unclear about what my job is (O)	1	2	3	4	5
____ 5. I have differences of opinions with my supervisors (O)/(S)	1	2	3	4	5
____ 6. Others' demands for my time at work are in conflict with each other (O)	1	2	3	4	5
____ 7. I lack confidence in "management" (O)	1	2	3	4	5
____ 8. "Management" expects me to interrupt my work for new priorities (O)	1	2	3	4	5
____ 9. There is conflict between my unit and others I must work with (O)	1	2	3	4	5
____10. I only get feedback when my performance is unsatisfactory (S)	1	2	3	4	5
____11. Decisions or changes which affect me are made "above" without my knowledge or involvement (O)	1	2	3	4	5
____12. I have too much to do and too little time to do it (ST)	1	2	3	4	5
____13. I feel overqualified for the work I actually do (ST)	1	2	3	4	5
____14. I feel underqualified for the work I actually do (ST)	1	2	3	4	5

	NEVER	RARELY	SOMETIMES	OFTEN	ALWAYS
____15. The people I work with closely are trained in a different field than mine (O)	1	2	3	4	5
____16. I must go to other departments to get my job done (O)	1	2	3	4	5
____17. I have unsettled conflicts with people in my department (or family) (S)	1	2	3	4	5
____18. I have unsettled conflicts with other departments (O)/(S)	1	2	3	4	5
____19. I get little personal support from the people I work with (S)	1	2	3	4	5
____20. I spend my time "fighting fires" rather than working to a plan (O)	1	2	3	4	5
____21. I feel family pressure about long hours, weekend work, etc. (S)	1	2	3	4	5
____22. I have self-imposed demands to meet scheduled deadlines (ST)	1	2	3	4	5
____23. I have difficulty giving negative feedback to peers (S)	1	2	3	4	5
____24. I have difficulty giving negative feedback to subordinates (or children) (S)	1	2	3	4	5
____25. I have difficulty dealing with agressive people (S)	1	2	3	4	5
____26. I have difficulty dealing with passive people (S)	1	2	3	4	5
____27. Overlapping responsibilities cause me problems (O)	1	2	3	4	5
____28. I am uncomfortable arbitrating a conflict among my peers (S)	1	2	3	4	5
____29. I am uncomfortable arbitrating a conflict among my subordinates (or children) (S)	1	2	3	4	5
____30. I avoid conflicts with peers (S)	1	2	3	4	5
____31. I avoid conflicts with superiors (S)	1	2	3	4	5
____32. I avoid conflicts with subordinates (S)	1	2	3	4	5
____33. Allocation of resources generates conflict in my organization (O)	1	2	3	4	5
____34. I experience frustration with conflicting procedures (O)	1	2	3	4	5
____35. My personal needs are in conflict with the organization (O)/(ST)	1	2	3	4	5
____36. I am bothered by my noisy environment (P)	1	2	3	4	5
____37. I have difficulty staying focused on a task (ST)	1	2	3	4	5
____38. My wife (husband) makes too many demands on me (S)	1	2	3	4	5
____39. I have concern over my parents' health (S)	1	2	3	4	5
____40. I have difficulty communicating with my children (S)	1	2	3	4	5
____41. I have difficulty saying what I feel (ST)	1	2	3	4	5

STRESS CYCLE AND INTERVENTIONS

The following is a diagram of the way we conceptualize stressors, stress and the effects of stress.

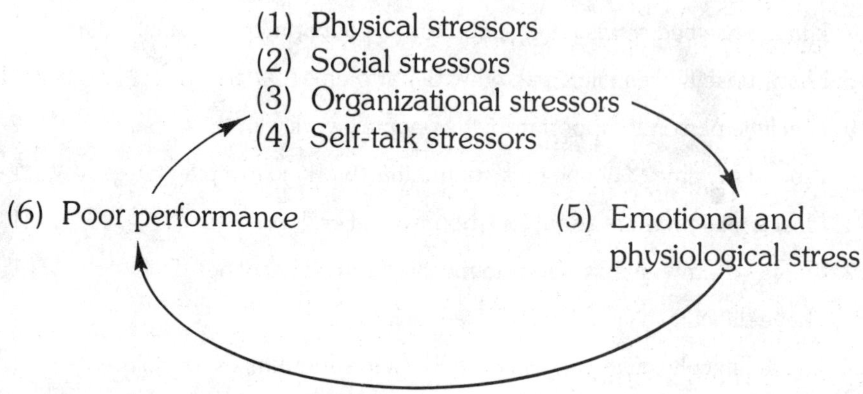

As you can see, there is a cyclical manner in which stress develops, manifests itself physiologically, and ultimately results in poor performance on the job, school, or in personal situations.

Some stressors come from the physical environment. These include such things as a small working space, no windows in a working area, a hot, sticky room or a room that is too cold, and traffic jams and slow elevators when you are in a hurry. These types of examples are labeled *"physical-environmental stressors."*

There are other factors, such as "social stressors," that can also begin a stress cycle. Examples of stressful social situations are: angry or aggressive people, having to give or receive negative feedback (such as a performance evaluation, or criticizing a colleague), and dealing with people who have difficulty expressing themselves or stating their needs. For those of you who work in service industries, examples might be very ill people or ungrateful clients.

Another category of stressors are *"organizational stressors."* Typical are such conditions as a lack of clear priorities as to work objectives, conflict between units or departments, or time pressure from work deadlines. All organizational stressors are not in the workplace. Families are themselves organizations, and various family roles may cause conflict. Educational institutions represent another group of organizations with role-related stress.

In addition to external factors, and probably our most common contributor to stress, is "self-talk." This refers to the self-imposed demands we place on ourselves in the form of "shoulds," "musts," "ought to's," and our own professional and personal "myths" or performance expectations. For example, many women suffer from the myth of the "perfect wife" or "perfect mother," while at the same time expecting to be the "perfect employee."

Actually, expecting to be the "perfect" anything can only lead to chronic dissatisfaction with one's performance, generating such self-talk as: "I'll never be able to please them," "I really should be pleasant to everyone," "I should do a better job," etc. These "verbal scripts" or self-dialogues are personal stressors, that, either by themselves or in combination with physical-environmental stressors, social stressors or organizational stressors, can lead to physiological and emotional stress—which is the next step in the stress cycle.

Physiological stress is manifested in such things as fatigue, tension in the back of the neck or shoulders, headaches, an upset stomach, and the multitude of physiological feelings we may have after a stressful situation. Emotional stress is present in feelings such as frustration, impatience and worry.

When we do not feel good, when we are in state of physiological stress, we do not do the job as well as we might if we were feeling fine. Therefore, as we move along the cycle, the physiological and emotional stresses cause poor performance on the job and/or at home. This poor performance can be manifested by losing our tempers, blaming others, taking it out on our families, or by simply not doing something as well as we usually do.

If we are not doing what we expect of ourselves, more negative self-talk results —which again can be a stressor for us. The cycle continues as we become a stressor to ourselves and/or to someone else (which may begin the cycle for them). Unless we do something to intervene in the cycle, it can snowball, fester and lower our effectiveness on a continuing basis.

You will learn certain skills in this program which you can apply at appropriate times to intervene in the stress cycle. Often, *physical-environmental stressors* cannot be avoided—you're stuck in a traffic jam and that's that. But you can use a breathing exercise to alleviate the full brunt of the stressful situation. You can also try imagery exercises—imagining you are in much more pleasant surroundings.

Assertion training has been found to be highly effective for *social stressors*, particularly in reducing stress from angry or aggressive people, or in dealing with difficult interpersonal situations. Also, active listening—rather than reacting—can help you deal more effectively with other people who are themselves under stress. Active listening can help you stay out of someone else's stress cycle.

Negative self-talk can be handled by cognitive restructuring—changing your myths and belief system to be more rational and more realistic, and thus easier on yourself. If you always expect perfection from yourself and do not always achieve it, you need to learn a new way to talk to yourself.

Organizational stressors may require intervention at many different levels, perhaps with respect to interpersonal communication, where changes can be made in relationships, but also in situations where the organization itself cannot be changed. None of us has enough power to change everything that bothers us in organizations (even in our own family). Thus, stress management in regard to organizational stressors may be utilized either to effectively change some of those stressors, or to cope with them if they cannot be changed.

If all, or any, of these stressors lead to physiological stress, relaxation exercises can help in minimizing the effects of both the physiological and the emotional stress. You cannot be relaxed and stressed at the same time.

If the cycle progresses to the point of poor performance, you may need to re-evaluate where the stress exists for you and what intervention is appropriate. All of these techniques should be integral parts of a complete stress management program; and all, combined or singly, can be effective in reducing and handling stress. The key is to know which are appropriate for you at various points in your stress cycle, and how to "plug in" the intervention effectively.

Exercise I-2

The purpose of this exercise is to look at your stress cycle. Some of the stressors should be taken from your stress questionnaire, and any that you marked "4 or 5" should be noted.

I. Either from the questionnaire or from other personal experiences, list three physical-environmental stressors:

A. ______

B. ______

C. ______

II. Also from the questionnaire or from your personal experience, list three social stressors:

A. ______

B. ______

C. ______

III. Organizational stressors?

A. ______

B. ______

C. ______

IV. In terms of negative self-talk and your job or family, please fill in the blank:

A. "I never ______

B. "I should ______

V. In terms of negative self-talk and your personal and social life, fill in the blank:

A. "I never ______

B. "I should ______

VI. Either from the questionnaire or your own experience, list your main three symptoms of physiological stress.

A. ______________________________

B. ______________________________

C. ______________________________

VII. Either from the questionnaire or your own experience, list your three main symptoms of emotional stress.

A. ______________________________

B. ______________________________

C. ______________________________

VIII. Either from the questionnaire or your own experience, list your main three behavior symptoms (poor performance).

A. ______________________________

B. ______________________________

C. ______________________________

Exercise I-3

Now you have defined your own stress cycle, and you may be interested in what you can do about it. Let us look first at the interventions you utilize now.

Either from the questionnaire or your personal experience, list your four most common methods for relaxing.

1. ______________________________

2. ______________________________

3. ______________________________

4. ______________________________

As mentioned above, interventions we propose are relaxation exercises, active listening, assertion training, learning to deal with aggressive or passive people, giving and receiving negative feedback, and cognitive restructuring . We will begin with relaxation, as it is totally in your control and does not require another person. Also, it is beneficial in dealing both with stressors, of all types, and with the resultant stress. After that we will discuss cognitive restructuring; it too is something you can do by yourself, for yourself. Also, its effects generalize into other types of stressors and stress. Although it is most helpful in terms of negative self-talk, it is very useful in assessing the importance of social and organizational stressors.

The third intervention will be active listening. This and the next one, assertion training, are most beneficial in dealing with social stressors but also are effective with organizational stressors. Finally, we will work with negative feedback, also effective for dealing with aggressive people and helpful in improving poor performance.

The most effective intervention is one that uses the techniques appropriately and in combination. Research has shown that changing the way you interact with others changes the way you talk to yourself and, therefore, the way you feel.

Exercise I-4

STRESS CYCLE INTERVENTIONS

A. List an intervention that would be appropriate for physical-environmental stressors:

____

B. List an intervention that would be appropriate for social stressors:

____

Any other? ______________________________

C. List an appropriate intervention for organizational stressors:

____

D. For negative self-talk?

____

E. Physiological stress can be dealt with by the following intervention:

____

F. If I reach the poor performance stage of the Stress Cycle I can utilize:

____

II

Relaxation Exercises

RELAXATION EXERCISES have two general purposes. One is to reduce or prevent the physical symptoms of stress; relaxation is an effective coping technique in situations that are stressful and cannot be changed. The second reason for teaching relaxation techniques is that some of us become so anxious in thinking about or approaching certain situations that we are unable to employ other techniques (e.g., cognitive restructuring) until our anxiety is reduced to a more manageable level. You should try these exercises at separate times, to learn which are the most effective for you.

BREATHING PATTERN

Controlling your breathing, or breathing in a special way for a few minutes, is often in and of itself an effective way to relax. Breathing exercises are commonly used in yoga and meditation, as well as in some natural childbirth techniques. Breathing that involves a long, slow exhalation is relaxing (for example, when you "sigh"). When you take in air, your diaphragm has to expand, thus tensing. As you let the air out, or exhale, it relaxes. So one way to relax is to spend more time exhaling. The diaphragmatic breathing not only encourages you to use your full capacity for breathing, but it also emphasizes a long, slow exhalation— and thus relaxation.

Many times, when people tense up, they breathe more rapidly and shallowly. The breathing exercise counteracts this pattern and also gets people to slow down, a first step in relaxing and gaining control. Breathing can be used alone or in combination with other relaxation exercises, such as progressive muscle relaxation and visualization techniques. Some people find it helpful to imagine all of their tension "flowing out" as they exhale.

As the breathing exercise is practiced in combination with muscle tensing and relaxing, it can become an effective "cue" for letting go of all your muscle tension. That is, it may become possible to simply breathe in deeply, breathe out, and automatically relax any or all of your muscles. It thus serves as a quick and convenient way to relax.

Breathing for relaxation, rather than utilizing about half of the time of the breathing cycle in inhalation and the other half in exhalation, is more effective if you attempt to break each breathing cycle into the following equally divided segments of time:

1. During segment one, inhale. (This should not be a deep inhalation, but only slightly deeper than your regular inhalation.)

   The goal is to breathe in your usual amount of air, but in a shorter period of time. Check that your stomach expands during this inhalation.

2. During segment two, begin to exhale. This should begin immediately upon completion of the inhalation. It should also be at a rate that allows you to continue to exhale comfortably for a few seconds.
3. During segment three, continue to relax. Attempt to focus on any awareness of relaxation that may spread across your chest area.
4. During segment four, complete the exhalation phase of the breathing cycle. Don't attempt to exhale all your air to a degree where you must tighten muscles to keep from expelling more than a comfortable amount.

   Again, during this segment, attempt to focus on awareness of relaxation.

A good way to practice this breathing is to use it several times throughout the day. Just remind yourself every hour or so to slow down and breathe this way for one or two minutes—it does not take much time, and you do not have to stop any other activity to do it. After practicing the breathing often enough, it can become an "automatic" type of response to stressful situations.

PROGRESSIVE MUSCLE RELAXATION

Progressive muscle relaxation, first presented by Dr. Joseph Wolpe, is a technique aimed at: a) creating an awareness of tension and relaxation, discovering which muscle groups express tension, and b) teaching a way to relax all of the muscles. It is called "progressive" because it proceeds through all of the major muscle groups, relaxing them one at a time, and eventually leads to total muscle relaxation.

Progressive relaxation can be utilized to relax completely or to relax only certain muscles. For example, people who work at a desk for several hours a day find it helpful to do a neck or shoulder exercise to loosen up those particular muscles when they have become stiff. Another advantage of learning progressive muscle relaxation is that it helps one become aware of when a single muscle starts to tighten up. Many times people become tense without knowing it, until they have a headache, backache, or neckache. By becoming more keenly aware of when and where the tension starts, many conditions like headaches can be totally avoided. It is much better to relax a neck muscle for a few minutes than to suffer through a painful headache for hours.

These exercises should be practiced (at least at first) in a quiet, comfortable place, reclining or even stretched out on the floor. Eventually you can learn to do certain parts, such as the neck and shoulder exercises, in your work situation, without doing the entire set.

You should spend 15-20 minutes doing these exercises, including the breathing. Going too fast is not conducive to relaxing.

Doing the breathing with the exercises accomplishes two things:

1. It allows a longer period of time for the relaxing portion of the exercise.
2. It conditions you to relax your muscles while you are exhaling. The ultimate goal of muscle relaxation is to be able to drop the muscle tensing portion of the exercise and to simply relax your various muscles as you exhale.

It must be reiterated that relaxation is a skill and has to be practiced. And, like any other skill, if it is let go too long, it can become rusty. Even people who become quite competent at relaxation need to give themselves a "booster" every so often. There are times when you may have to review by first tensing a muscle and then relaxing again. However, after it has been learned the first time, relaxation will come faster and easier.

The following instructions are best read by someone else or put on a tape by you and played on a recorder.

First, take three slow deep breaths . .
Close your eyes when you feel comfortable...
Inhale and exhale, long and slow.
Try to focus on your body and on letting the tension "flow out" as you exhale...

Relaxation of Arms

(Time: 4-5 minutes)

Settle back as comfortably as you can and let yourself relax to the best of your ability.
Now, as you relax, clench your right fist.
Clench it tighter and tighter, and study the tension as you do so.
Keep it clenched and feel the tension in your right fist, hand and forearm.
Now relax...
Let the fingers of your right hand become loose...
Observe the contrast in your feelings.

Now, let yourself go and try to become more relaxed all over.
Once more, clench your right fist really tight.
Hold it, and notice the tension again.
Now, let go, relax, let your fingers straighten out...
Notice the difference once more.

Now repeat that with your left fist.
Clench your left fist while the rest of your body relaxes.
Clench that fist tighter and feel the tension.
And now relax... Again, enjoy the contrast.
Repeat that once more, clench the left fist, tight and tense.
Now do the opposite of tension—relax and feel the difference...
Continue relaxing like that for awhile.

Clench both fists tighter and tighter, both fists tense, forearms tense.
Study the sensations... and relax...
Straighten out your fingers and feel that relaxation...
Continue relaxing your hands and forearms more and more.

Now bend your elbows and tense your biceps.
Tense them harder and study the tension feeling.
All right, straighten out your arms...
Let them relax and feel the difference again...
Let the relaxation develop.
Once more, tense your biceps.
Hold the tension and observe it carefully.
Straighten the arms and relax...
Relax to the best of your ability...
Each time pay close attention to your feelings when you tense up and when you relax...

Now straighten your arms, straighten them so that you feel most tension in the triceps muscles along the back of your arms.
Stretch your arms and feel the tension.
And now relax...
Get your arms back into a comfortable position...
Let the relaxation proceed on its own...
The arms should feel comfortably heavy as you allow them to relax.
Straighten the arms once more so that you feel the tension in the triceps muscles.
Feel that tension... and relax.
Now let's concentrate on pure relaxation in the arms without any tension...
Get your arms comfortable and let them relax further and further...
Continue relaxing your arms ever further...
Even when your arms seem fully relaxed, try to go that extra bit further...
Try to achieve deeper and deeper levels of relaxation.

Relaxation of Facial Area with Neck, Shoulders, and Upper Back

(Time: 4-5 minutes)

Let all your muscles go loose and heavy.
Just settle back quietly and comfortably.
Wrinkle up your forehead now, wrinkle it tighter.
And now stop wrinkling up your forehead.
Relax and smooth it out...
Picture the entire forehead and scalp becoming smoother, as the relaxation increases...
Now frown and crease your brows and study the tension.
Let go of the tension again...
Smooth out the forehead once more.
Now, close your eyes.
Keep your eyes closed, gently, comfortably, and notice the relaxation.

Now clench your jaws, push your teeth together.
Study the tension throughout the jaws.
Relax your jaws now...
Let your lips part slightly...
Appreciate the relaxation.
Now press your tongue hard against the roof of your mouth.
Look for the tension.
All right, let your tongue return to a comfortable and relaxed position.
Now purse your lips, press your lips together tighter and tighter.
Relax the lips...
Notice the contrast between tension and relaxation...
Feel the relaxation all over your face, all over your forehead, and scalp, eyes, jaws, lips, tongue, and throat...
The relaxation progresses further and further.

Now attend to your neck muscles.
Press your head back as far as it can go and feel the tension in the neck.
Roll it to the right and feel the tension shift...
Now roll it to the left.
Straighten your head and bring it forward.
Press your chin against your chest.
Let your head return to a comfortable position and study the relaxation...
Let the relaxation develop.

Shrug your shoulders right up.
Hold the tension.
Drop your shoulders and feel the relaxation...
Neck and shoulders relaxed.
Shrug your shoulders again and move them around.
Bring your shoulders up and forward and back.
Feel the tension in your shoulders and in your upper back.
Drop your shoulders once more and relax...
Let the relaxation spread deep into the shoulders right into your back muscles.
Relax your neck and throat, and your jaws and other facial areas, as the pure relaxation takes over and grows deeper... deeper... even deeper.

Relaxation of Chest, Stomach, and Lower Back

(Time: 4-5 minutes)

Relax your entire body to the best of your ability.
Feel that comfortable heaviness that accompanies relaxation.
Breathe easily and freely in and out…
Notice how the relaxation increases as you exhale…
As you breathe out, just feel that relaxation.
Now breathe right in and fill your lungs.
Inhale deeply and hold your breath.
Study the tension.
Now exhale, let the walls of your chest grow loose, and push the air out automatically…
Continue relaxing and breathe freely and gently…
Feel the relaxation and enjoy it.

With the rest of your body as relaxed as possible, fill your lungs again.
Breathe in deeply and hold it again.
Now breathe out and appreciate the relief, just breathe normally…
Continue relaxing your chest and let the relaxation spread to your back, shoulders, neck and arms…
Merely let go and enjoy the relaxation.

Now let's pay attention to your abdominal muscles, your stomach area.
Tighten your stomach muscles, make your abdomen hard.
Notice the tension.
And relax, let the muscles loosen and notice the contrast.
Once more, press and tighten your stomach muscles.
Hold the tension and study it.
And relax, notice the general well-being that comes with relaxing your stomach.
Now draw your stomach in.
Pull the muscles right in and feel the tension this way.
Now relax again… Let your stomach out…
Continue breathing normally and easily and feel the gentle massaging action all over your chest and stomach.

Now pull your stomach in again and hold the tension.
Once more pull in and feel the tension.

Now relax your stomach fully...
Let the tension dissolve as the relaxation grows deeper.
Each time you breathe out, notice the rhythmic relaxation both in your lungs and in your stomach...
Notice how your chest and your stomach relax more and more...
Try and let go of all contractions anywhere in your body.

Now direct your attention to your lower back.
Arch up your back, make your lower back quite hollow, and feel the tension along your spine.
Now settle down comfortably again, relaxing the lower back.
Just arch your back up and feel the tensions as you do so.
Try to keep the rest of your body as relaxed as possible.
Try to localize the tension throughout your lower back area.
Relax once more, relaxing further and further...
Relax your lower back, relax your upper back, spread the relaxation to your stomach, chest, shoulders, arms and facial area...
These parts relaxing further and further and further and even deeper.

Relaxation of Hips, Thighs and Calves followed by complete body relaxation

(Time: 4-5 minutes)

Let go of all tensions and relax.
Now flex your buttocks and thighs.
Flex your thighs by pressing down your heels as hard as you can.
Relax and notice the difference.
Straighten your knees and flex your thigh muscles again.
Hold the tension.
Relax your hips and thighs...
Allow the relaxation to proceed on its own.

Press your feet and toes downwards, away from your face, so that your calf muscles become tense.
Study that tension.
Relax your feet and calves.
This time, bend your feet towards your face so that you feel tension along your shins.
Bring your toes right up.
Relax again... Keep relaxing for awhile...
Now let yourself relax further all over...
Relax your feet, ankles, calves and shins, knees, thighs, buttocks and hips...
Feel the heaviness of your lower body as you relax still further.
Now spread the relaxation to your stomach, waist and lower back.
Let go more and more deeply...
Make sure no tension has crept into your throat.
Relax your neck and your jaws and all your facial muscles.
Keep relaxing your whole body like that for awhile...
Let yourself relax.
Now you can become twice as relaxed as you are merely by taking in a really deep breath and slowly exhaling, with your eyes closed, so that you become less aware of objects and movements around you, and thus prevent any surface tensions from developing.
Breathe in deeply and feel yourself becoming heavier.
Take in a long, deep breath and exhale very slowly...
Feel how heavy and relaxed you have become.

In a state of perfect relaxation, you should feel unwilling to move a single muscle in your body.

Think about the effort that would be required to raise your right arm.
As you think about that, see if you can notice any tensions that might have crept into your shoulders and arm.
Now you decide not to lift the arm, but to continue relaxing...
Observe the relief and the disappearance of the tension.
Just carry on, relaxing like that... Continue relaxing...
When you wish to get up, count backwards from four to one.
You should now feel fine and refreshed, wide awake and calm.

CHECKLIST VERSION OF PROGRESSIVE MUSCLE RELAXATION EXERCISES

Tense a muscle first, then relax it. Notice the contrast between the feelings of tension in a muscle and relaxation of that muscle. Try *inhaling* as you tense a muscle and *exhaling* as you relax it. Spend more time relaxing than tensing. Eventually, the tensing portion can be dropped.

1. FISTS—Clench right fist, then left, then both.
2. BICEPS—Bend elbows, tense biceps
3. TRICEPS—Straighten and feel tension along back of arms
4. FOREHEAD—Wrinkle forehead, frown
5. EYES—Close tightly
6. JAWS—Clench jaw, bite teeth together
7. TONGUE—Press against roof of mouth
8. LIPS—Press together
9. NECK—Press your head back as far as it will go—roll to right, roll to left, bring head forward to chest
10. SHOULDERS—Shrug one, and then the other, and then both
11. CHEST—Fill lungs with air, hold, and breathe out
12. STOMACH—Tighten stomach muscles—draw stomach out
13. LOWER BACK—Arch up back, make lower back hollow, feel tension along spine
14. BUTTOCKS AND THIGHS—Flex by pressing down on heels; then straighten knees and flex again
15. CALVES—Press feet and toes downwards, tensing calf muscles
16. ANKLES AND SHINS—Bend feet toward head, feeling tension along shins

Exercise II-1

In what muscle groups did you feel a little extra tension, a sense of familiarity? You have experienced *that* tension before frequently.

A. ____

B. ____

C. ____

These are the groups of muscles to practice tensing *and* relaxing several times during the day.

AUTOGENIC TRAINING

"Autogenic" is a word that means self-generating or self-moving. It refers to a process whereby people can relax by giving themselves verbal cues for relaxation. It is thought to facilitate the body's "homeostatic" mechanism — a self-balancing of sorts. This is, of course, a goal of all of the relaxation techniques. When people become too tense, they can bring themselves back into balance by relaxing.

For our purpose here, we will be using one of the autogenic exercises — the heaviness series. It consists of simply saying (silently) a series of phrases to oneself. For example, "my right arm is heavy," or "my left arm is heavy," etc. The most important thing to remember is that it does not matter whether you really feel heavy or not. And this brings up a concept that is central to all of relaxation. That concept is called "passive concentration."

Although it sounds at first like a contradictory term, it can best be understood by looking at the difference between "active" and "passive" concentration. In the exercise described above, it makes a great deal of difference if instead of saying "my right arm is heavy," you say "I want my right arm to be heavy." This second phrase is active concentration. It is goal-directed activity. It is almost like saying "I am going to make myself relax, or else!", which certainly is not relaxation producing. It is trying to force something instead of simply letting go.

So, how does one passively concentrate? It is done by saying a phrase like "my right arm is heavy," slowly and repeatedly, and knowing that it does not matter if you feel heavy. There are many sensations that occur with relaxation, like feeling lighter, or heavier. Many people feel a tingling or warmth. You may even feel nothing at all. But you can still be relaxed.

The word "heavy" was chosen for this particular exercise because it has been found that heaviness is often associated with relaxation, and that it seemed to facilitate relaxation when people used it, even though a variety of other sensations often occurred at the same time. Most important is simply not to expect anything, but just allow your body to relax.

It is very important to include a "termination" process at the end of each heaviness exercise. This process consists of flexing your arms, taking a deep breath, and opening your eyes. This is done to reactivate the system or allow it to adjust gradually to a higher state of arousal, one that is needed for getting up and walking around.

Generally, the heaviness exercise takes only about two minutes to complete. However, most people like to spend 15 or 20 minutes and do several. It is an exercise that can be extremely helpful for people who have difficulties falling asleep. In instances where you are using the exercise to fall asleep, you do not need to go through the termination process, since you do not want to reactivate your system.

This exercise can be done sitting in a chair, as we will do here, or lying down on a couch, bed, or floor. As with the other exercises, the more it is practiced, the easier it will be to quickly reach a state of complete relaxation. Here again, it is best to tape this ahead or to have someone else read the instructions.

Autogenic Exercises

1. HEAVINESS EXERCISE

   (Repeat each phrase slowly three times.)
   "My right arm is heavy.
   My left arm is heavy.
   Both my arms are heavy.
   My right leg is heavy.
   My left leg is heavy
   Both my legs are heavy.
   (Optional)—My neck and shoulders are heavy."

2. WARMTH EXERCISE

   (For those wishing an additional autogenic exercise)
   "My right arm is heavy.
   My arms and legs are heavy.
   My right arm is warm.
   My left arm is warm.
   Both my arms are warm.
   My right leg is warm.
   My left leg is warm.
   Both my legs are warm.
   My arms and legs are warm.

Termination (After Exercise)

3. CALMING EXERCISE (short version).

   Begin by breathing slowly with a longer exhale than inhale, and on the inhale saying, "I am," and on the exhale saying, "calm."

   Repeat ten times.

   (Instead of "calm," "serene," "relaxed," and "one" have been used effectively.)

VISUALIZATION

Visualization or imagery is another technique often used for relaxation. It is a sort of day-dreaming for relaxation purposes: a specific scene is imagined, like lying on the grass in the warm sun, and then it is developed. That is, you continue to picture yourself in that scene, noticing how it feels to be "lying in the grass, feeling the warmth of the sun, feeling a soft breeze," etc. You do this until you feel very relaxed, just as you would if you really were lying in the grass.

This is the last relaxation exercise to be introduced, and you may want to begin by taking about 3-5 minutes to relax yourself with one of the other exercises before attempting to visualize. Then the leader (or taped version) can guide you through one or more visualizations. After this is done, silently create your own picture, visualize it for 2-3 minutes, and time your breathing slowly.

SAMPLE VISUALIZATIONS

1. It is very early in the morning as you wake up. You feel nice and warm under the covers. It is very quiet in the house—so quiet, you know that no one else is up yet. You are the only one awake. You can almost "hear" the quiet. It is so peaceful, and you feel very cozy in bed, just listening to the quiet. (variation) You wake up to hear it raining softly on the roof. It looks cold and wet outside. Inside you are nice and dry and warm under the covers... etc.

2. You're lying on the beach, warm under the sun. The sand feels nice and soft underneath you. You're very calm and relaxed, almost falling asleep. You can hear the waves rolling in, gently. You feel so comfortable ... (variation) You're lying on the grass in the park. The sun makes you feel nice and warm and comfortable—sort of sleepy. You can hear the birds in the trees. You can hear the soft rustling of leaves in the trees and feel a slight breeze, making it relaxing and comfortable ... etc.

3. You are walking slowly through a beautiful green forest. The only sounds you can hear are the sounds of the birds in the distance. It is very quiet here, and you continue to walk slowly and quietly, enjoying the calm and peacefulness. It is a warm day, but the forest is slightly cool, making you feel very comfortable, just the right temperature. You have the forest all to yourself with nothing to disturb you, just feeling good, feeling calm and relaxed.

4. You are sitting on a bank at the side of a lake. The water is very still and quite clear. The lake is flat and shiny. If you look into the distance you can see the water sparkling from the sun shining on it. It is very comfortable where you're sitting, and you find it so easy to relax just gazing out at the lake. (variation) It is summer time and nice and warm outside. You are just about to go into the water (i.e., pool or lake) with your raft. You slide into the cool, calm, water and then onto your raft. You lie on your back on the raft and just float there. You let your arms and legs dangle in the cool water as you're floating. You relax completely just letting your raft hold you up. It is very comfortable. You lie that way for a long time, feeling relaxed...

Exercise II-2

A. Which of the exercises were the most effective for you?

B. Can you think of any combinations of the exercises that might work for you?

III

Cognitive Restructuring

(CHANGING THE WAY THAT YOU THINK, OR THE ROTO-ROOTER OF THE MIND)

MANY OF US THINK that other people and the events in our lives cause us to feel the way that we do. Thus, we often blame things *external* to us for feelings of stress and emotional upset. In doing this, however, we often neglect an important factor not only in the *cause* of stress, but in the management of stress. That factor is the way that we *think,* or "talk to ourselves," about the events in our lives. It is the point we have labeled "self-talk" on the Stress Cycle. This chapter will present a method called "cognitive restructuring" for constructively dealing with feelings of stress that arise from the irrational or faulty thinking that we all engage in from time to time.

Before presenting this method, however, it is first necessary to consider the relationship between thoughts, feelings and behavior.

THE STRUCTURE OF EMOTIONAL RESPONSES

The A-B-C's Model

Many people think that thoughts, feelings and behavior are separate and distinct categories. You often hear people say things such as: "I have a gut-level feeling about this," or "I can't help the way I feel—it just happens." This assumes that thoughts and feelings occur independently and are not directly related. However, quite the opposite is true. Rarely does a feeling "just happen," and you *do* have the capability to change the way that you feel.

One model for examining the relationship between thoughts, feelings and behaviors was developed by Dr. Albert Ellis: the A-B-C model.

Point A in the ABC framework refers to the activating event. For example, your boss might reprimand you for failing to complete a project on time. Following this, you feel upset or nervous about your work-performance. Point C represents your feelings about the event. It also includes your *behavior.* For example, you might, upon being criticized, become defensive and retort back with: "Well, what do you think I am—a work horse?" Many people mistakenly believe that Point A—the event—leads directly to Point C—feelings and behavior:

A ACTIVATING EVENT
(Boss's reprimand)
↓
C FEELINGS AND BEHAVIOR
(upset, nervous, defensive)

So it is the *boss* that makes *you* upset. After all, he did reprimand you, didn't he?

Something very important, however, occurs between A and C; and indeed, produces C. That something is Point B, our self-talk, and that self-talk influences our feelings and behavior.

A ACTIVATING EVENT
(Boss's reprimand)

↓

B YOUR THINKING
("I forgot all about it—I should be fired")

↓

C FEELINGS AND BEHAVIORS
(upset, nervous, defensive)

Now we can see that the boss does begin the process, but that it is *your* own thinking that produces your feelings. The self-talk can be rational or irrational, functional or dysfunctional. Since even the best of us make errors and are unable to live up to our self-expectations, it is important to look at the sources of Point B, and our most common self-statements. These self-statements can become habitual responses to stress, like smoking or drinking coffee, and need to be changed—just like other undesirable habits. A different example of self-talk on your part would be:

A ACTIVATING EVENT
(Boss's reprimand)

↓

B YOUR THINKING
("I wish I had finished on time, but I didn't.")

↓

C FEELINGS AND BEHAVIOR
(Disappointment—but kept in perspective: "I generally do better.")

Thus, one event can be perceived in a variety of ways and can result in a number of different emotional responses. It is not the stress event that makes you tense, but how you think of the event. Often our feelings of stress rise from thinking that is incorrect or irrational. For example, if our internal self-talk about failing at an attempted task is that it is not only unfortunate and inconvenient, but that it is *awful* and *catastrophic,* we are likely to experience feelings such as depression, anxiety, or tension. Similarly, feelings of anger and hostility usually develop if we believe that someone who acts unfairly *absolutely should not* act that way. This type of irrational thinking suggests that we have or should have control over another's behavior. Since we obviously do not, we are setting ourselves up for feeling stressed each time we have such thoughts.

While many people have been aware that thoughts somehow lead to feelings, few realize that they actually have the ability to change unwanted or irrational thoughts voluntarily to result in different emotional feelings. Such change is possible through a process called "cognitive restructuring." Basically, what this means is that we can learn by practicing specific "coping skills" to restructure our thoughts, reduce stress, and increase relatively positive or neutral feelings.

Exercise III-1

1. Is it the *facts and events* in our lives that upset us and lead to stress or the *view* that we take of them? Explain and give an example.

____

2. Do feelings always arise from within, or can other people *make us feel* a certain way? Explain.

____

3. Where do feelings come from?

____

4. How are our thoughts important in leading to our emotional responses?

____

5. Feelings of stress often arise from ______________________ thinking.

6. What is cognitive restructuring?

____

7. How can we use cognitive restructuring to reduce stress and alter unwanted emotional responses?

____

8. Fill in the outline below describing the A-B-C theory of human behavior.

A. ____

B. ____

C. ____

9. Think of the last time you were feeling a strong, unpleasant emotion. Write that emotion under C in the following diagram. Now, under A, write in the event that happened before the emotion occurred. Finally, under B, put your best guess as to what you were thinking between the event and the emotion. Was your thinking rational? Was it functional, i.e., did it help you?

A ACTIVATING EVENT

____

____

____

____

____

B YOUR THINKING

____

____

____

____

____

C FEELINGS AND BEHAVIOR

____

____

____

____

____

ROLE MYTHS

One powerful and pervasive source of our self-talk or inner dialogue is the myths associated with the various roles that we play. These myths relate to being "perfect" in these roles and are often in conflict with each other. Thus, a most common contributor to stress is negative self-talk which refers to self-imposed demands—the need to appear perfect to ourselves or others in all of our many roles.

For instance, you are a mother as well as a nurse in a hospital which is understaffed. One morning your child awakens with a high fever. If you leave your child with a babysitter and go to work, you are certainly not living up to the myth of the perfect mother. If, on the other hand, you stay home with your child and do not go to work when you know they are understaffed, you are certainly not the perfect nurse.

For another example, one of the authors is a wife, mother, administrator, psychologist, teacher, female role model — not to mention daughter, friend, runner and mentor. In all of these roles, she really wants to be superwoman, and she used to berate herself when she could not quite pull it off all the time. Let us look at some of the perfection she was seeking in these familial and professional roles.

MYTHS OF THE PERFECT WIFE

1. Always responds to her husband's needs
2. Lives for his successes
3. Always knows *what* he wants for dinner and *when* he wants to eat
4. Always finds his boss charming even when he isn't
5. Puts her husband's career ahead of her own

MYTHS OF THE PERFECT PSYCHOLOGIST

1. Loves *all* people
2. Is always delighted to be awakened in the middle of the night by someone who "just wants to talk"
3. Has her own personal life in perfect order
4. Has perfect children

MYTHS OF THE PERFECT ADMINISTRATOR

1. Always fair
2. Always available
3. Can always bend the rules for *you*
4. Has a secret source of resources

MYTHS OF THE PERFECT RUNNER

1. Eats only health foods
2. Always has a spiritual experience while running
3. Loves all other joggers
4. Fights creeping narcissism

Another of the authors shares some of the same myths but has another compelling one:

MYTHS OF THE PERFECT NURSE

1. Cares deeply for all patients
2. Has no life aside from serving mankind
3. Considers herself the physician's handmaiden
4. Never makes an error
5. Is compulsively neat

You get the idea. Striving for perfection in all of these roles may be worthy, but it is stressful. There are times when it just will not work.

Exercise III-2

(a) List your major roles, in descending order of their importance to you. (Some may be the same as those we have listed above; others will be different.)

ROLES

1. ______________________
2. ______________________
3. ______________________
4. ______________________
5. ______________________
6. ______________________

(b) Now, with respect to each of the first three, the ones you assigned highest priority, list *your* major role myths.

1. ROLE NO. 1 ______________________

MAJOR MYTHS

a. ______________________

b. ______________________

c. ______________________

d. ______________________

e. ______________________

2. ROLE NO. 2 ______________________

MAJOR MYTHS

a. ______________________

b. ______________________

c. ______________________

d. ______________________

e. ______________________

3. ROLE NO. 3 ______________________________

MAJOR MYTHS

a. ______________________________

b. ______________________________

c. ______________________________

d. ______________________________

e. ______________________________

(c) Look over your myths. Which ones pose conflicts (such as the example of the mother and nurse)?

1. ______________ and ______________

2. ______________ and ______________

3. ______________ and ______________

We will come back to this later. The point is that a balanced and rational approach is necessary to manage the stress produced by the conflicted roles and our own striving for perfection.

In addition to the role myths, we also have some beliefs which have some very illogical, irrational bases. These beliefs generate the irrational thoughts we described earlier. The basis of the beliefs is that if things do not work out as well as expected, it is catastrophic. Common examples are:

1. If I don't have love or approval from the people I want to love and approve of me, I'm worthless.
2. If other people don't appreciate my help, that just shows they're ungrateful.
3. If I don't achieve up to my full potential, that just shows I'm a worthless slob.
4. If I find myself getting angry, that just shows I'm losing ground.
5. If I go off my diet, that proves I don't have any will power.
6. My way is the only right, just and rational way to do things.
7. If I don't like everybody I work with, that just shows I'm uncaring.
8. If I don't preoccupy myself with a threatening situation, I won't be able to handle it.
9. If I'm not thoroughly competent, adequate and achieving, I have no value in this society.
10. My past is all-important and explanatory; therefore I can't help some of the things I do.

One way to relieve our stress is to question such habitual, irrational beliefs. But first you have to recognize that you subscribe to them.

Exercise III-3

Go back over the list of irrational beliefs and circle the ones that you hold personally.

Now return to the earlier A-B-C example you wrote in at the end of Exercise III-1 and write an irrational belief around the Activating Event (A).

Next, return to your role myths that you listed in Exercise III-2 and write your irrational beliefs about each of the roles (e.g., If I am not the first in my class, that just proves I should not be in graduate school).

1. Role: ____________________

   Belief: ____________________

2. Role: ____________________

   Belief: ____________________

3. Role: ____________________

   Belief: ____________________

RATIONAL SELF-ANALYSIS

After analyzing our irrational beliefs and resultant illogical thoughts, it is time to begin to change them. It must be recognized, however, that we are all human beings; and, therefore, no one is rational all of the time. The first step in this change process is to establish some criteria for differentiating between rational and irrational beliefs. These are some which have been found to be useful:

1. Are the beliefs based on *objective* reality? That is, would a mixed group of people all agree that the event happened in the way you perceived it? Or, do you exaggerate and personalize experiences?

2. Are they helpful to you?
   Self-destructive thoughts are usually irrational.

3. Are they useful in reducing conflicts with other people?
   Or, do you set up a me vs. them situation?

4. Do they help you reach your short and long term goals, or do they get in the way?

5. Do they reduce emotional conflict? That is, do they help you feel the way you want to feel, or do they help you feel miserable?

DOING A RATIONAL ANALYSIS

Using the real-life situation that you described in earlier exercises, or another which has occurred to you, write down under A below the facts and events of the situation as *you perceive them.* (Do not attempt to correct any inaccurate perceptions at this time. For example, A might initially read, "my thoughtless boss yelled at me today." Since the word "thoughtless" is an opinion or evaluation, the actual event is more realistically, "my boss yelled at me today." However, these changes are more appropriately made later.) Next, write in at C the way you felt, e.g., tense, angry, depressed. It is important here to identify and eliminate from this section *thoughts* that are sometimes disguised as *feelings,* e.g., "I feel stupid and irresponsible," or "I feel as if you're being inconsiderate."

The next step is to write down in the B section the thoughts or self-talk that come to mind as you think about the situation. You may find this somewhat difficult, because it separates your thoughts from your feelings and requires recognition of how thoughts logically lead to emotional responses, but learning to do this is the point of the exercise; we hope we have convinced you that it can be done.

A ACTIVATING EVENT

____

____

____

____

____

↓

B YOUR THINKING

____

____

____

____

____

↓

C FEELINGS AND BEHAVIOR

____

____

____

____

____

Now is the time to go back and examine the accuracy of your *perception* of the event—by analyzing the accuracy of the facts and events written into the A section. Write this objective version in D below. A rule of thumb to apply here is: If you can record the event on a mechanical recording device, i.e., a camera or a tape recorder, it is probably a fact. If the event cannot be recorded mechanically, it is probably an opinion, a feeling, or an evaluation. The example given earlier illustrates this point: the statement "my *thoughtless* boss yelled at me today" does not pass this examination, because the event cannot be recorded mechanically. Only that part of the event that *can* be recorded ("my boss yelled at me today") goes into the D section. This should help you see how misperceptions of situations can alter your internal dialogue and affect your emotional response.

(At this point, check back and apply the five criteria of objectivity to each thought in B section to determine whether or not it is rational. Now it should be clear which of your thoughts are irrational, leading to negative emotional feelings, and which are not.)

Now decide how you would like to feel in the situation you described in D, and enter the feeling under F. It is often unrealistic to want to have a *positive* emotional response to a stressful situation. It is usually more realistic and appropriate to desire a relatively neutral emotional feeling (e.g., calm).

You can now address the E section and develop *rational alternatives* to the *irrational thoughts* you had in B. The rational alternatives must be personally acceptable to you, and they should meet at least three of the five criteria for rational thinking. It must also be emphasized that recognizing a thought to be irrational does not automatically suggest what *is* rational. Finally, it is important to emphasize that writing this in this format is only a practice exercise for undertaking a rational plan of action and changing unwanted feelings and behaviors.

D OBJECTIVE EVENTS

____

____

____

____

____

E YOUR RATIONAL THOUGHTS

____

____

____

____

____

F DESIRED FEELINGS AND BEHAVIOR

____

____

____

____

____

Here is another example from one of the authors' experiences:

A ACTIVATING EVENT
A staff member does not take good advice which I gave her.

↓

B MY THINKING
1. Maybe I came on too strong.
2. I probably gave her bad advice.
3. She does not know what is good for her.

↓

C FEELINGS AND BEHAVIOR
1. Self-doubts about leadership.
2. Avoid person.

This could be redone in the following manner.

D OBJECTIVE EVENT
Staff member did not do what I suggested.

↓

E MY RATIONAL THINKING
She is responsible for her own behavior.

↓

F DESIRED FEELING OR BEHAVIOR
Relaxed with continued pleasant interactions.

Exercise III-4

Choose another situation which has led to unpleasant feelings in the past and go through the same analysis.

A ACTIVATING EVENT

____

____

____

____

____

↓

B YOUR THINKING

____

____

____

____

____

↓

C FEELINGS AND BEHAVIOR

____

____

____

____

____

Review the criteria that distinguishes between rational and irrational thinking and continue.

D OBJECTIVE EVENT

E YOUR RATIONAL THINKING

F YOUR DESIRED FEELINGS AND BEHAVIOR

The more you practice the analysis of your thoughts and making them more rational, the better you will feel. Remember: *Your thoughts control your feelings.*

COGNITIVE RESTRUCTURING

Integration

Recognizing that the way we *think* determines the way we *feel* is the most important message in this chapter. Attending to our inner dialogue (sometimes called our own "B-grade movie") requires some changes in our usual way of dealing with ourselves and our interactions.

When we look at our role myths, we recognize that we chose many of the roles we occupy because of the myths. Maybe you decide to become a teacher because you really like the idea of molding young minds and "producing the citizens of tomorrow." But when one of your students is caught stealing hubcaps, both *you* and the *community* judge you in terms of the myths. The point is that we tend to reinforce each other in maintaining our myths. We want our nurses to be more loving, our psychologists more caring, our doctors more perfect—than is humanly possible.

A way to balance our thoughts and feelings is to maintain a high standard for ourselves but know that we will not always be able to meet it. When we are not perfect, that does not mean we fail.

For example, the following irrational belief is a very common one for people in our working environment.

> *"If everyone who I feel is important does not like what I'm doing, then I must be a failure."*

This belief supports a number of our role myths and leads to feelings of self-doubt. We can change (restructure) this belief to make it easier to achieve:

> *"It would be nice to be respected and loved by everyone, but I am not worthless when I do not achieve this goal."*

Thus, we retain a standard which is high, but we recognize that we will not always attain it.

Exercise III-5

Return to the irrational beliefs that you circled earlier. Write down one of them.

Belief: ____

____

____

____

Write down as many reasons as you can why this belief is irrational. In the example presented above, for instance, the word "everyone" should be challenged. Also, we cannot control others' approval of us, only our own. How many reasons can you find to refute the belief you wrote down?

Challenge: ____

____

____

____

Now, rewrite the belief to one which is more reasonable.

New Belief: ____

____

____

____

Pick one more for practice.

Belief: ____

____

____

____

Challenge: ____

____

____

____

New Belief: ____

____

____

____

We have presented the basic skills necessary for cognitive restructuring. Only your practice with them will make them a part of your new thinking and therefore give you more positive, or at least neutral, feelings.

IV

Active Listening

THE FIRST TWO INTERVENTIONS we have discussed are ones you can do by yourself, without anyone else being involved. Learning relaxation skills and ways of changing our self-talk is a logical way to begin, as we are the ones who are in control of those processes (although they often feel out of control). On the other hand, active listening is an intervention which addresses our interaction with others.

As you look back over your stress questionnaire, note the social stressors. Active listening, and the subsequent assertiveness training, are two very effective ways of dealing with these stressors.

One of the authors was yelled at by an angry physician. She said to the physician, "You sound angry. Are you just angry, or are you angry at me?" The physician replied, "I'm angry at not having a piece of equipment I need. I'm not angry at you, but thanks for asking."

Thus we are introduced to one of the simplest, yet most effective tools for reducing stress — active listening. It is almost too simple to be true. And, the effects of its use are multiple.

First of all, it is a defusing device: it defuses anger simply because of the acknowledgment from one person to another that yes, he *is* angry. Second, it clarifies where, in fact, that anger is directed. Is it a personal, vindictive anger? Or is someone mad about an inanimate object, and not actually *towards* another person, like the physician in the example above. Third, and probably most important when we are talking about stress reduction, active listening allows you to decide whether or not you want to "buy into" someone else's momentary craziness; it buys time, allowing you to conserve time and energy with opening statements that *acknowledge* someone else's anger, frustration, annoyances, whatever, but preserving your *option* of participating or not participating in those annoyances. Let's go back to the beginning and set the stage for all of this.

In any given situation, whether the situation is stressful or not, there are three parts to the communication process. There is always (1) a sender of the message, (2) a receiver of the message and (3) the content of the material. The message can be either verbal or nonverbal.

When all three parts of the communication process are functioning smoothly, effective communication takes place, and there is little room for misunderstanding. However, if one or more of the three parts are not functioning correctly—either the sender, receiver or message—incomplete or inappropriate messages may be relayed, with a resulting increase in stress levels and misunderstanding. For example, if the sender of the message has had a bad day and is feeling thoroughly frustrated, that person might say "I can't stand it here any longer!" The receiver of the message, perhaps a co-worker who feels taken aback by the outburst, could take the exclamation personally and think "My gosh, what did I do? Is she angry with me, or just plain angry?"

Active listening is an excellent method of checking out those assumptions; it is a legitimate way of breaking the emotional chain—that could evolve with a reply of, "I can't stand it here either, and your frustration and outburst are *really* making me even more uptight." Such a reply could cloud or even mistakenly crystallize the content of the message "I can't stand it here" and leave room for highly emotional and highly stressful communication.

Let's suggest an Active Listening answer instead. "I can't stand it here any longer!" warrants the reply "you sound upset about your work"—a brief, simple reply that acknowledges the other person's feeling, gives the active listener a chance to hear more about how the person is *actually* feeling, and allows the listener the option of either continuing with the conversation or leaving it with a simple acknowledgment. To continue on, the active listening script in this case could run like this:

Sender: "I can't stand this place any more!"

Receiver: "You sound really upset about your work."

Sender: "You're darn right I'm upset. I get no feedback, either positive or negative about how I'm doing and I don't feel appreciated."

Receiver: "Well I am sorry you're upset, but I wanted to check out with you to see if you were upset at me or simply at work."

The conversation could either continue from here into a problem-solving session for the sender, or it could terminate. But, what has taken place is at least a defusing of emotions—both the sender's and the receiver's. The receiver has delayed responding with his feelings and thereby has had the opportunity to verify any underlying messages, feelings and emotions of the sender before developing a personal view of the situation and its effect on his (the receiver's) own behavior. The usual result of an active listening reply is that the sender cools down, and the situation is placed in a more rational and reasonable perspective, both for the sender and for the receiver.

Magic? Not really, but almost. However, some techniques are necessary for it all to work smoothly. These techniques are largely based on one idea: that the receiver, in responding to a highly charged, emotional statement should remember to *avoid,* at first, being any of the following toward the sender: rationalizing, questioning, supporting, defending, judging, or parroting. What do we mean by each of these?

Rationalizing: Adding your reasons for the other person feeling the way she does. For example:

Sender: "All I ever get to do is the scut work around here. I feel as though I'm xeroxing my life away."

Receiver (rationalizing): "Oh, come on now, it's just a really hot day, and you're just in a bad mood."

This answer may or may not be true, but it doesn't allow any verification of the original message and the original emotion of the message.

Questioning: Questioning the motive or reasoning of the sender in his/her original message. For example:

Sender (muttering under his breath): "You know, you can't trust anyone around here without getting stabbed in the back."

Receiver (questioning): "Oh really, who are you talking about? Anyone I know?"

This reply allows the original message to either fester and get worse, or to get lost in a sea of gossip, without any resolution of the issue.

Supporting: Now, this is a difficult one to avoid, because it is in most of our natures, particularly in the helping professions, to help and support one another. But once again, what we are proposing here is that you allow the sender to verbalize the message, then allow yourself to verify the content, and, most important, give yourself time to decide whether or not you want to or can help. Supporting is admirable, but in terms of stress reduction, namely your own, and in terms of being rational about the "myth of the perfect helping professional," you may need to assess the situation with an active listening technique rather than being immediately supportive. For example:

Sender: "I could die here, and no one would even notice."

Receiver (supporting): "Now, now, it's o.k. It's all going to be better. I will help you."

This reply may not have acknowledged the content or emotion of the original statement and may get you involved in a situation you wished you had avoided.

Defending: Defending occurs when the receiver backs up the apparent purpose of the message without further information, or on the other hand is defensive in response to the sender. For example:

Sender (in a loud voice): "I've been working on this report for the last three days, and now you send this other memo telling me I have to add this, delete that, and change something else."

Receiver (defensive): "The memo is important. I wrote it, and I am the only one who knows the whole picture. No more discussion."

This reply just leads to escalation of stress for both of you.

Judging: Making a judgement about the motive, personality or reasoning of the sender about her message. For example:

Sender: "Well, I'm supposed to get up in front of the group with my presentation today. I've written and rewritten my material, but I'm sure they won't like it. They'll probably laugh me off the podium."

Receiver: "You shouldn't feel that way."

This answer is a sure way of telling the sender you're just not interested, and that you know how she *should* feel.

Parroting: Parroting is simply and obnoxiously restating exactly what it was the other person said.

Sender: "Gee, this place is really disgusting."

Receiver: "Sounds like you think this place is really disgusting."

A reply such as this provides virtually no acknowledgment of the intent or reasoning behind the message.

Assuming then that rationalizing, questioning, supporting, defending, judging and parroting should be avoided, what do we propose? That a very simple active listening technique be employed as the *first* reply. The technique is simple and almost like filling in a blank. It is, in a sense, being a "mirror" to the speaker regarding what he has said (but without simply parroting).

The idea of active listening was first proposed by psychologist Carl Rogers. The format is simple:

"You sound ___________ about ___________________________."

angry	this
upset	that
worried	the other thing

Let's go back to some of our examples, and try this technique.

Sender: "All I ever get to do is the scut work around here. I feel as though I'm xeroxing my life away."

Receiver: "You sound *really frustrated* about *your work*."

or

Sender: "You know, you can't trust anyone around here without getting stabbed in the back."

Receiver: "You sound *like you're not sure* of *what's really happening* at work."

or

Sender: "I could die here, and no one would even notice."

Receiver: "You sound really *upset*."

An easy way to remember the important elements in an active listening situation is to try to recall the characteristics of an exchange where you felt free to really talk about feelings and about the things that concerned you. Think about the characteristics of the social climate and of the person you were speaking with. Some of the elements may include:

1. Understanding
2. Warmth and acceptance
3. Nonevaluation
4. Equality
5. Freedom
6. Faith in your ability to solve your problems.

The active listener is reflective and empathic, in order that the sender may feel accepted and understood. The active listener is objective and nonjudgemental, to avoid clouding the issue with feelings of guilt and inferiority. By identifying the feelings being transmitted, the active listener is essentially telling the sender he is free to express his emotions. By clarifying the direction of these feelings, the active listener is promoting the problem-solving process, and the sender becomes more assured of his abilities to handle emotional situations.

Of course, any new technique such as active listening may require a change in the way you generally respond to a message. Like most behavioral change, it will probably require practice.

Exercise IV-1

In each of the following situations, fill in a receiver's active listening response.

(a) Sender: (a co-worker): "I have worked my fingers to the bone and have received nothing in return."

Receiver: ______________________________

(b) Sender (a child): "You couldn't understand me. You're too old."

Receiver: ______________________________

(c) Sender (a doctor on a unit): "This place is a mess. It really takes the cake as the number one pig pen in this hospital."

Receiver: ______________________________

(d) Sender (a patient with a complaint): "Damn administrators. Don't you have any appreciation for the families of sick people?"

Receiver: ______________________________

(e) Sender: "Why do you always say 'uh-huh' to me?"

Receiver: ______________________________

(f) Sender (wife and husband): "All I ever do is try to talk to children who whine. I feel whiney myself."

Receiver: ______________________________

Some sample replies:

(a) "You really sound angry about not getting that raise."
(b) "You really sound angry about something." Then, if the child answers "yes," you have the option of saying, "Do you want to tell me about it?"
(c) "It sounds like you're upset about the equipment in the hall."
(d) "You sound frustrated about your treatment.'
(e) "You sound like you don't think I'm really acknowledging you."
(f) "You sound mad about something. Are you mad at me, or did you have a bad day?"

"You sound like, you sound like," may seem repetitious, and certainly other responses can be used, such as, "it appears," or "it seems like." But, whatever language you may choose, there is much more effective and clear communication as a result.

To sum up: By employing active listening skills, the receiver promotes effective communication by:

1. **Clarifying the content of the communication.** The first step in communication is to understand what is being said.
2. **Verifying nonverbal messages.** The receiver needs to check out the consistency of body language and tone of voice with the verbal communication. An active listening response can help you verify what is *not* being said as well as what *is* being said.
3. **Gathering additional information.** Clarifying verbal and nonverbal messages and verifying the feelings of the speaker allows the receiver an opportunity to learn more and to better interpret the interaction before developing her personal view.
4. **Providing a genuine personal response.** Active listening promotes understanding and acceptance, clarifying both thoughts and emotions.
5. **Promoting problem-solving behavior.** Once the sender's feelings have been identified, the interaction can be directed towards objective problem-solving.

Once again, the technique of active listening allows the receiver to play an active role in the interaction without having to commit personal feelings or thoughts regarding either the sender or the content. This is an excellent stress reducer, because it allows you to conserve your time and energy with a simple statement such as "you sound like...," before you decide that you want to involve yourself in what is going on. And, by maintaining an objective stance, the active listener encourages a sharing of ideas and paves the way for a freer exchange of other points of view. It can work. It *does* work.

Exercise IV-2

Look at the situations that cause you stress. Do you feel overwhelmed and unsure about what to say? Either passive or aggressive verbal behavior can cause us stress. Think of three times when you felt upset when someone spoke to you. Write your responses to each one as you remember it. Then construct an active listening response.

1. Sender: ______________________________

   Your response then: ______________________________

   An active listening response: ______________________________

2. Sender: ______________________________

   Your response then: ______________________________

   An active listening response: ______________________________

3. Sender: ______________________________

Your response then: ____

____

____

An active listening response: ____

____

____

Exercise IV-3

1. Name three parts to the communication process.
   a. ______________________________
   b. ______________________________
   c. ______________________________

2. List three advantages of using active listening in reducing stress.
   a. ______________________________
   b. ______________________________
   c. ______________________________

3. Name six techniques to *avoid* when considering an active listening response.
   a. ______________________________
   b. ______________________________
   c. ______________________________
   d. ______________________________
   e. ______________________________
   f. ______________________________

4. List the characteristics of effective communication through active listening.

a. ______________________________

b. ______________________________

c. ______________________________

d. ______________________________

e. ______________________________

f. ______________________________

ANSWERS

1. Three parts to the communication process:
   a. Sender
   b. Receiver
   c. Message

2. Three advantages of using active listening in reducing stress:
   a. The receiver can be active without committing a personal response.
   b. The active listener can portray or "mirror" the other's feelings and thoughts.
   c. The technique refocuses attention back to clarification of the content.

3. Six techniques to avoid when considering an active listening response:
   a. Rationalizing
   b. Questioning
   c. Supporting
   d. Defending
   e. Judging
   f. Parroting

4. The characteristics of effective communication through active listening:
   a. Understanding
   b. Acceptance and warmth
   c. Nonevaluative and nonjudgemental
   d. Equality
   e. Freedom
   f. Faith in an individual's ability to solve his own problems

V

Assertion Training

ONE OF THE MOST COMMON sources of stress is not being able to tell someone else what we are feeling and thinking. When you took the stress questionnaire, you may have checked one of the following items:

"I have differences of opinion with my supervisors."
"I have difficulty giving negative feedback to peers."
"I have difficulty giving negative feedback to subordinates."
"I have difficulty dealing with aggressive people."
"I have difficulty dealing with passive people."
"I avoid conflicts with peers or superiors or subordinates."
"I have unsettled conflicts with people in my department."

If you did check some of these, you are affected by social stressors. Social stressors come, for the most part, from difficult interpersonal interactions — interactions where we are not able to express ourselves appropriately or effectively, and as a result feel angry at the other person or ourselves for holding "it" in or inappropriately blurting "it" out. "It" refers to the statements we wished we had said, if we had only been "true" to ourselves and had had the self-confidence to state, diplomatically but firmly, what we believe.

The active listening skills discussed in the preceding chapter certainly help in terms of recognizing what is occuring in a situation and what the other person is experiencing. Now, with assertion training, it is your turn to express yourself in a way that helps you get your needs met and makes you feel better about yourself and, therefore, less stressed.

For instance, in the example given earlier of your boss catching you in an error, you may feel angry at being discovered to be imperfect. Hopefully, you will use an active listening response (after taking a deep breath) like "you sound upset with me." Then you may want to make a positive statement such as "I feel badly, too, and I will correct it as soon as possible." This is less stressful than feeling guilty, angry, clamming up, or becoming vengeful. To be assertive is to say what you mean in a straightforward way without demeaning someone else.

For another example, one of the authors was kept waiting by a dentist recently. First, he was late in seeing her and then, while she was imprisoned in the chair, he left her for a ten-minute phone call. She told his assistant (in a level voice) that if he did not begin work by 8:50, she would have to leave, as she would be keeping other people waiting at her office. He returned at 8:47, and she said to him, "If you cannot start working on my teeth within three minutes, I have to leave. I won't leave angry, but I will leave." The dentist got right to work, continued without interruption *and* remained pleasant.

There are times when you want to tell people how you feel, what you think is important, and what you can and can't do. You want to tell them that you have listened to them, but that you cannot do what they want. You want to tell them what irritates or doesn't irritate you, and how you work best or how you don't. And, you want to do this in a way that is accepted by other people, and in a way in which you get your point across effectively. It doesn't do you any good to yell or to have people guess what your needs are. Chances are they will guess wrong, and your needs, as a result, will not be met. It also doesn't do too much good to hope that if you are "nice" to people, they will somehow know what it is you need and give it to you. This doesn't work too well.

Assertion is "owning" what you need, including your emotions, and not putting the responsibility for that ownership on someone else. Assertion is also talking about things in such a way that people will listen and not be offended, and giving them the opportunity to respond in return. Assertion is a combination of many things. It is a manner of acting and reacting in an appropriately honest manner that is direct, self-respecting, self-expressing and straightforward. It is a behavior that instills self-confidence, that is goal oriented (but not at the expense of others), and is defined by above-board negotiation where yours and others' rights are respected.

It sounds like the "perfect" way of behaving. But, as we all know, there is no "perfect" behavior; nor is there such a thing as an assertive pill which we swallow and makes us instantaneously assertive. Assertion is, however, integral to self-esteem and, as such, helps in innumerable interpersonal situations where being direct, honest, and straightforward is a ticket to better interactions.

Like all learned behaviors, assertion needs to be practiced. Part of that practice is differentiating it from two opposing behavior styles: passive and aggressive.

At one time or another we all manifest these three behavior styles—passive, assertive and aggressive. We are assertive with certain people and in certain situations, and passive or aggressive in other situations. Being passive or aggressive may get you what you want for a short period of time, but after that, people start avoiding you. In order not to have people avoid you, let's define what we mean by passive and what we mean by aggressive.

When we are passive, we allow other people to choose for us. We are usually emotionally dishonest, indirect and self-denying. This often leads to anger, for while the passive person is denying himself things, he is usually "keeping score" of all that he misses, and at some point, his gunnysack blows up. "Gunnysacking" means that a person is packing away in a mythical "sack" all of those things that anger him but that he doesn't express. He tells you everything is "just fine," but underneath he is seething, and the "sack" can blow up at the slightest provocation.

For instance, imagine this scenario: You are in an office situation, and you ask a passive person to catch the telephones while you and the rest of the staff go out for a birthday lunch. "That will be just fine," the person replies, angry that she was not included but feeling too emotional to say anything. Whomp ... that anger gets put into the sack. Next, you ask her to do a mail run because you are unable to get to the mail room that day. "That will be just fine," and whomp ... anger at being asked to do something else gets put into the sack. The requests and the same replies go on until finally you ask the passive person to sharpen a pencil, and the person blows up for "no apparent reason." The sack had gotten so full it had burst.

The passive person is very concerned about concealing anger he can feel welling up inside. When he thinks he is controlling it, it actually controls him; for as he gets more and more angry, he approaches the point where he has to explode. And when he does explode, it is usually out of all proportion to what really occurred.

Passive people generally are burdened with myths, such as the myth of the "perfect wife," "nurse," "mother," "provider." And part of that myth is that they never get angry. But, at the same time they are saying to themselves, "it isn't fair."

Being passive may be a behavior of choice at times (e.g., when you simply want to get rid of someone, you may choose to discourage the development of a relationship by acting passive). But, for the most part, being passive doesn't get your needs met, and it does not help other people to know what in the world to do with you. There is an underlying belief system for the passive person which says, "I should never make anyone uncomfortable or displeased, except myself." It is very difficult to deal with passive people, because they aren't really "straight" with you. They are masters of the surprise attack and, all in all, they are like "pinning jello to the wall." Just when you think you know where they are, the slipping begins.

At the opposite end of the scale is the aggressive person. Aggressive people like to have an inordinate amount of control of themselves and everyone else. They like to choose for others and are inappropriately honest to the point of being tactless. The directness is usually only for their own self-enhancement. When we are aggressive we often say, "Well, at least they know where I stand." They do, and in no uncertain terms. When aggressive, we involve ourselves in win-lose situations in which only we can win. The aggressive person usually achieves her goal, but at others' expense. Her rights are upheld, but if you are on the receiving end, yours are violated.

The underlying belief system is, "I have to put others down in order to protect myself." Aggressive people want control, and compared to the passive person, at least they are straightforward about it. But, in getting that control, the aggressive person wants to take control of others, and as a result, the other person in the interaction feels humiliated, defensive, resentful and usually hurt. Sound familiar? It is no fun dealing with the aggressive person who is adept at stepping on toes in the process of getting his needs met.

One easy way to show the difference between being passive, assertive and aggressive is to practice what you consider first a passive, then an assertive and finally an aggressive handshake on another person. (Eye contact and handshakes are probably the two primary means of labeling people when we first meet them.) Feel the difference as you try each of the three handshakes. Which do you prefer?

We are advocating assertion as the optimum way of behaving in most circumstances. However, there is a difference that needs to be pointed out here—a difference between assertive choice and assertive behavior. Assertive behavior is connected with rights, self-esteem, and getting one's needs met. But, it may be more appropriate at one time or another to behave non-assertively if you foresee a better outcome through another type of behavior. If behaving assertively means getting fired, and this is not an appropriate alternative, be non-assertive for a more desired result.

Assertive choice is linked to "ourselves and the circumstances we find ourselves in." Behaviors vary depending on the individual and the circumstances. What at one time may be an assertive choice, may not be the best choice at a later time. Assertive choice means that one has control and has the choice to be more assertive or non-assertive in a given situation. For example, you are standing in a supermarket line, and a very large person cuts in front of you. Your assertive remark would be, "I would appreciate it if you would go to the back of the line." However, a more realistic approach might be to not make waves, in the cause of self-preservation. Hence, assertive choice does not involve "shoulds." (e.g., "You *should* be assertive all the time.") Assertive choice gives you options. It is a common error to try to be assertive in all situations without analyzing the alternatives.

Exercise V-1

Read the Comparison of Alternative Behavior Styles below and circle any items which describe you. Are you more often assertive, aggressive or passive?

COMPARISON OF ALTERNATIVE BEHAVIOR STYLES

	Passive	Assertive	Aggressive
CHARACTERISTICS	Allow others to choose for you. Emotionally dishonest. Indirect, self-denying, inhibited. In win-lose situations you lose. If you do get your own way, it is indirect.	Choose for self. Appropriately honest. Direct, self-respecting, self-expressing, straightforward. Convert win-lose to win-win.	Choose for others. Inappropriately honest (tactless). Direct, self-enhancing. Self-expressive, derogatory. Win-lose situation which you win.
YOUR OWN FEELINGS ON THE EXCHANGE	Anxious, ignored, helpless, manipulated. Angry at yourself and/or others.	Confident, self-respecting, goal oriented, valued. Later: accomplished.	Righteous, superior, depreciatory, controlling Later: possibly guilty.
OTHERS' FEELINGS IN THE EXCHANGE	Guilty or superior. Frustrated with you.	Valued, respected.	Humiliated, defensive resentful, hurt.
OTHERS' VIEW OF YOU IN THE EXCHANGE	Lack of respect. Distrust. Can be considered a pushover. Do not know where you stand.	Respect, trust, know where you stand.	Vengeful, angry, distrustful, fearful.
OUTCOME	Others achieve their goals at your expense. Your rights are violated.	Outcome determined by above-board negotiation. Your and others' rights respected.	You achieve your goal at others' expense. Your rights upheld; others violated.
UNDERLYING BELIEF SYSTEM	I should never make anyone uncomfortable or displeased ... except myself.	I have a responsibility to protect my own rights: I respect others but not necessarily their behavior.	I have to put others down to protect myself.

How do you know an assertive person when you see one? There are both non-verbal and verbal cues. The first non-verbal cue is eye contact. The assertive person uses direct eye contact. This doesn't mean staring someone down and not blinking, it only means looking the other person in the eye when you are speaking to her and holding the contact fairly steadily throughout the conversation. When you conclude what you have to say, that last instant of contact serves as a period.

The second non-verbal cue is the use of hand gestures. Gestures are most effective when they help emphasize the content and importance of what you say. This does not mean allowing your hands to wildly gesticulate all over. This is particularly important if you are a smoker. Busy, smoking hands are a distraction. Posture can also indicate assertiveness: sitting or standing straight, not hunched over, and not hiding in the corner of a room. Projecting one's voice, not yelling, but speaking up and not mumbling is being assertive. It is common to see people make an assertive comment and then ruin the effect by dropping or raising their voice at the end. For example, in a parent role, you might say in a firm voice, "I want you to clean your room immediately." By itself that sounds good, but then instead of waiting for a response, you say, "Okay?"

Other phrases which can detract from assertiveness (particularly when delivered in a whiney or reedy voice) are, "You know?", or "You know what I mean." Being assertive involves knowing when to stop talking.

One hallmark of assertive behavior is making "I" statements, such as "I feel, I like, I wish, I would appreciate, I need." The passive person puts responsibility on someone else and usually says "don't you think that?" (Which really means "I think" without taking responsibility.) On the other hand, the aggressive person takes that privilege away from you and states, "you ought not to do this."

"I" statements take responsibility for our decision making. We often refuse to take that responsibility and keep from saying what we mean. This may be from a myth about obligation: if I tell you what I need, you are going to feel obligated to do it. Making "I" statements doesn't obligate another person to respond in a certain way. Only he is responsible for his emotions and behavior. It is *our* responsibility to state what our preferences are.

Other hallmarks of being assertive include the use of short sentences and creating pauses, if necessary, to make sure the other person understands what you are saying. If your sentences are too long, you lose people. And, as you have probably noticed, long rambling statements on any subject are an indication of either aggressive or passive behavior. In either case, the speaker appears to be afraid to stop talking.

Exercise V-2

One way to practice these techniques of assertive behavior is to talk about trivial topics and to receive feedback on your:

eye contact
hand gestures
posture
voice firmness
"I" statements
short sentences
pauses for other persons' feedback

The two purposes of this exercise are (1) to practice assertive behaviors with content that is not anxiety provoking, and (2) to build confidence in being able to make "small talk" effectively. Trivial subjects we often use for practice are: lint, bacon grease and army boots. Try them or another of your choice. When you realize you have something to say on *any* subject, you begin feeling more confident about meeting strangers and conversing with them.

Fill out the following:

Trivial subjects I discussed ________________________________

Feedback I received on my:

Eye contact ____

____

Hand gestures ____

____

Posture ____

____

Voice firmness ____

____

"I" statements ____

____

Short sentences ____

____

Pauses for feedback ____

Learning to be assertive and practicing a new type of behavior often creates anxiety for people. Assertiveness seems overwhelming if you have spent years feeling guilty when you say "no," making "you" statements ("don't *you* think we should go the movies?"), instead of "I" statements ("I would really like to go to the movies."), and shirking in corners instead of placing yourself in a more conspicuous place in a room. Assertiveness needs to be practiced in order for you to feel comfortable using it. And , at first it may seem unnatural. A wise sage once said, "Everything worth doing, is worth doing badly at first." Most people will not notice if you are not perfectly assertive all at once.

Sometimes anxiety about the new behavior gets to the point where it can actually "block" an assertive response, or make it extremely uncomfortable for you. You can learn to manage such anxiety through a variety of techniques such as the relaxation training described earlier.

Anxiety, however, can seem overwhelming in certain circumstances, making you forget all about being assertive and instead revert back to passive or aggressive reactions. For example, if someone comes into the room where you are sitting right now and yells, "This place is a mess!", could you automatically respond with an assertive statement? Or, how would you feel if you were asked to get up on your chair and tell about your most embarrassing moment to a group of about 30 people? Assertive? Probably not. Anxious? Probably so.

One way of measuring such anxiety is through a technique called SUDS. No, it has nothing to do with washing; it stands for Subjective Units of Discomfort Scale. (Wolpe, 1973) It is in fact a scale useful in quantitatively measuring anxiety levels. If you can learn to put a number on your anxiety, behaviors leading to that anxiety and the anxiety itself can be more specifically pinpointed.

The SUDS scale runs from zero to one hundred. If your SUDS level is between zero and 30, you are extremely relaxed, to the point of probably being asleep. If your SUDS level is from 30 to 75, you are probably active and productive. Between the range 75 and 100 you are probably "distressed" to the point of not being productive and being very uncomfortable. For example, performance evaluations instill SUDS levels of about 80-90 in most employees. Being asked for your opinion in a group meeting may raise your SUDS level to about 99+. If you can learn to rate your anxiety, giving it a number, you can learn to reduce that number to a more manageable level through relaxation training, active listening and more assertive responses to anxiety-producing situations.

Assertive responses to anxiety-producing situations can be very effective to reduce SUDS levels. You can learn to manage stress by reducing SUDS and utilizing assertions as a means to this end. Through assertion you can reduce personal stress, by being more confident in your ability to deal with aggressive and passive people, reduce anger, and reduce anxiety (SUDS) about the possible negative consequence of an interaction. Assertion training is a skill that, if practiced and appropriately used, can allow you to express your thoughts, feelings and beliefs "in direct, honest, and appropriate ways which respect the rights of other people." (Lange and Jakubowski, 1976)

Social stressors and negative self-talk can also be handled in an effective way through assertion, thereby preventing or reducing the physiological stress and poor performance components of the stress cycle. Assertion will help you solve problems, get the results you want faster, and give you energy for the next task at hand. It is thus an important communications skill as well as an important stress reduction technique.

Exercise V-3

Subjective Units of Discomfort Scale (SUDS)

Remember the SUDS scale—

0 ⟵ practically asleep ⟶ 50 ⟵ active productive ⟶ 75 ⟵ tense ⟶ 100

Write down your SUDS level in response to the following situations:

You are asked to stand up in front of a group of 100 people and talk about the new project you've initiated at work. ______

You've just had a flat tire on a busy street after work, and a man has gotten out of his car to yell at you about blocking traffic. ______

You have to give a performance evaluation to an employee. ______

You have to get a performance evaluation from your supervisor. ______

You are about to be married. You are walking down the aisle, and you trip. ______

You are thinking about your schedule for next week. ______

You are just about to drop off to sleep. ______

You are drinking a glass of warm, mulled wine in front of the fire on a cold winter's eve. ______

You are working on a report that is really interesting, and you have given yourself a lot of time to complete it. ______

You are walking down the hall, and you see the person with whom you had a fight an hour earlier. ______

You are hiking in the woods on a lovely spring day. ______

Exercise V-4

(1) Write a short script on a situation which causes your SUDS level to go to 75 or above. (2) Try some problem-solving and ask yourself whether an assertive behavior response would help relieve your anxiety. (3) Write down what that response would be.

Situation:

Assertive response:

Exercise V-5

Areas to Work on

The "Areas to Work On" sheet, p. 87, is an excellent tool to encourage you to write down situations where you usually act in either a passive or aggressive manner and where you would rather act assertively. Like the preceding exercise, it can be used as a problem-solving sheet, where you look at the situations that are causing you SUDS levels over 75—and which have been going on for a long time and need to be resolved.

The sheet is simple to use. In each horizontal column, first briefly describe one of your common stressful situations, and then write down: (1) the people involved, such as "co-worker," "boss," "physician," or whoever it may be that causes the situation or causes your SUDS level to go up; (2) how you usually behave — what do you usually do in that situation that causes you to feel uncomfortable and to come away not feeling assertive but rather passive, aggressive, or as if you had been "had"; and (3) for the "Desired Behavior" portion of the sheet, how you would prefer to act—what would be your assertive response if you could magically produce it. (4) Then, give it all a number; put down your SUDS level when the situation is occurring.

Here is an example:

Situation	**People involved**	**Typical behavior**	**Desired behavior**	**SUDS**
Being yelled at in front of co-workers	Boss, me, co-workers	I become the "shrinking violet." Do nothing.	Speak to my boss in private about how his behavior affects me. Feel confident about doing so.	95

The most important part of this sheet is "Desired Behavior." In another chapter we will be talking about giving negative feedback and dealing with aggressive people. Both can be used in the above situation and can be effective stress management tools to reduce SUDS levels.

Using the Areas to Work On sheet is a very concrete first step in reacting with desired assertive behavior rather than with undesirable passive or aggressive behavior. If you define what the situation is that is bothering you, and write it down and give it a SUDS level, some resolution of that situation can begin to evolve. As a result, your stress level can begin to come down in response to the situation.

AREAS TO WORK ON

SITUATION	PEOPLE INVOLVED	TYPICAL BEHAVIOR/RESPONSE	DESIRED BEHAVIOR	PRESENT SUDS LEVEL

VI

Dealing with Aggressive People

DEALING WITH AGGRESSIVE people, like giving negative feedback (next chapter), is often an unpleasant task. The techniques presented in this chapter are intended for use when it has become impossible to communicate with another person on a calm or rational level because of their aggressive behavior and its effect on you.

Very few people other than prizefighters enjoy dealing with aggressive people. Many of us feel ineffective when we do encounter such people and often end up feeling angry and acting aggressive ourselves. It is very *natural* to react to an aggressive person by either fighting back or by attempting to placate him. Generally, nothing is solved by either of these behaviors. The aggressive person may be insecure and immature, and thus reacts to any challenge with increased aggression. On the other hand, if he is merely catered to or placated, his aggressiveness is only reinforced, and continues.

Since the aggressive person often sees other people as "the enemy," and continually violates the rights of others in attempting to "conquer" them, it seems clear that one needs to pay attention to one's *own* rights and needs when dealing with him. Generally, this involves clarifying the issue at hand and minimizing the amount of emotional "dumping" to which one is subjected. There are a number of ways to achieve this.

Sometimes it is possible to defuse the aggression by reflecting back the emotion expressed ("you sound *very angry* about that") and getting the person to define the actual issue. This is our now familiar Active Listening techique. At other times it is more difficult to deal with the aggressive person, who may continue to "rant and rave." One method for stopping a stream of anger is called the "broken record" technique. This involves formulating one statement and repeating it over and over again, not giving the person more information, but sticking to that one statement. (e.g., "I can't talk with you right now," or "I can't talk with you when you yell.") By doing this, you give the person no further incentive to fight, nor do you end up giving endless "explanations" or unnecessarily defending yourself.

It often helps to think of the other person's aggressive behavior as the "poorer performance" part of the stress cycle, and to realize that you were probably not the original stressor but are actually on the recycling end of something you did not begin.

If the aggressive person refuses to discontinue her tirade, it may be necessary to simply refuse to interact with her any longer, until she is willing to discuss things calmly and maturely. The method for this is called "shifting gears." This means deferring the conversation to another time, when the person (and possibly yourself) is not so angry or aggressive. This can be done by stating your opinion that the conversation is going nowhere and needs to be talked about at another time. ("Why don't we talk about this tomorrow at 10:00 when you (and I) are a little more calm." It may be easier to lead into this by saying "I am getting anxious (angry) and need to think about this some more."

Finally, there are some occasions when simply telling the person verbally that you do not wish to deal with his aggression is not enough. Then you may need the technique for getting your message across which is called "time out." You simply ignore the person by looking away or attending to other things, such as making out a "shopping list" in your head while sitting there. You just stop giving the person any forum for his aggression.

Exercise VI — *Dealing with Aggressive People*

Let us try out each of these techniques—broken record, shifting gears, and time out. Each is appropriate in different situations and in handling differing degrees of aggression.

Go back to your sheet on "Areas to Work On." Are there any situations you defined where the person you were dealing with was aggressive? If so, try writing out an appropriate broken record statement to such a situation, then a shifting gears statement, and finally, think about whether or not time out would be appropriate. For example, if a loud and demanding person came up to you insisting that a physician that he had an appointment with was late, and kept badgering you for information about when the physician would be available, you could reply with a broken record like "the doctor will be with you in just 5 minutes. I have spoken with him, and he will see you then."

If the persistently aggressive person keeps up the tirade, you can keep up the same broken record (not allowing the person any more informaion than that one statement)—or try out shifting gears: "I can't tell you anything more about the appointment. I'l get back to you in a few minutes if there are any changes, but I *will* get back to you." If none of your situations to work on involve dealing with aggressive people, try out the examples below. Write a broken record response or a shifting gears response to each aggressive statement:

1. "I told you I wanted some action on my bill right now!"

2. "What do you mean 'my car's not ready.' I brought it in at 8:00 this morning, and I need it now—and I mean now."

3. "Dinner's not cooked. The kids are out playing. The house looks like a pig pen. The dog's chewing up my shoes. What's going on here?"

4. "I'm sick of the insolent treatment I get around here. No one ever tells me what's going on or why."

5. "You really tick me off. I needed that report at 9:00, and it's not ready. You and your usual disorganized habits!"

VII

Giving and Receiving Negative Feedback

GIVING OR RECEIVING CRITICISM or negative feedback is often difficult for people, and is commonly avoided. It is one of the most frequently checked items on the stress questionnaire. In this section, you will learn a constructive approach to giving and receiving negative feedback—one that is actually stress reducing for all parties involved.

Thus far you have been exposed to a large amount of information regarding stressors, behavioral responses, and intervention techniques. Some will not be as useful for you as others. Not all stimuli in our environment affect all of us in the same way. It is equally true that not all stimuli affect any one person in the same way all of the time. Perhaps, in a few of the examples given throughout this manual that attempted to define a "stressful" situation, your response has been, "That isn't stressful at all for me."

There are a good many factors that influence the way in which a stimulus affects us, and these have been discussed in earlier chapters. In terms of negative feedback, however, there is an additional influencing factor that appears to play a major role in determining the manner with which we handle these types of situations. In most interactions that involve either giving or receiving negative feedback, the *emotional consequence* of that feedback assumes great importance. This consequence can be either real or imagined; but either way, it creates stress for most people.

In negative feedback situations we often become concerned either with how the other person will respond to receiving the comment, or with how the other person perceives us when we are giving it. Because the feedback is negative in nature, a fear develops that the other person will wind up feeling negative about himself or us. Most people don't want to make others feel that they are poorly thought of, and most people don't want to believe that others think poorly of them.

Picture yourself at work (or home) on a very busy day. There are quite alot of things you need to have completed before the end of the day. Unfortunately, you could get a bit more done if your co-worker (spouse) would only handle his share of the responsibilities. You know that this person doesn't mean for you to do extra work, but he is easily distracted and never quite finishes the task at hand. For your own mental and physical health, however, you decide that you need to present your thoughts and feelings to him to somehow alter the situation.

You suspect, and maybe even know, that your co-worker (spouse) will respond to this negative feedback by accusing you of calling him a lazy slob. You anticipate that the consequence of your interaction with him will be a confrontation regarding your opinion of him as a person. Now, you dread even bringing up the subject, because of the fear you have for an anticipated battle regarding feelings towards one another, and you contemplate not discussing it at all.

Now let's switch roles. Again, picture yourself at work (home) on a very busy day. Your boss (or spouse) walks into the room, and by looking at him you can tell that he is angry. He comes over to you and says in a rather loud voice, "You really made a mess of this job. Everything has been put in backwards; it will take twice as long now to correct it." Your immediate response is to think that your boss (or spouse) sees you as a real incompetent idiot. He must think you can never do anything right, and that makes you feel very bad. You want to say something, but the words don't come to mind. You imagine that the consequence of this exchange is that your boss (or spouse) feels you are an inferior human being.

Both of these examples demonstrate that the anticipated consequence of the interpersonal exchange is having an influence on the message being communicated. Without even establishing the validity of the negative feelings about themselves, the people in these situations are allowing these feelings to interfere with the communication process. The focus of the exchange is shifted from the negative feedback (message) to the personal feelings (emotional consequence).

Situations that involve having to share a negative comment about someone's behavior are uncomfortable for most people. This type of exchange may continue to be somewhat uncomfortable for you simply because of its negative nature. The important point to remember is that negative feedback, if clear and concise, can be a positive step towards solving the problem at hand. However, one must focus on the *message* being relayed and not on the anticipated *emotional consequence* of the exchange.

There are several steps that can be taken in the negative feedback process that may help to clarify the message you want to send. In addition, these steps will assist you in objectively viewing negative feedback as a recipient.

The first step in this process is to describe the situation clearly. You want to make objective notations regarding the circumstances that warrant negative feedback. In other words, take care to identify precisely the behavior—what the other person does, or doesn't do — that you would like to see changed. An example of this objective description might be: your co-worker leaves fifteen minutes early for lunch; you have to be responsible for all of the clean-up, and you don't have a backup available for last minute orders. The target behavior is leaving early.

While you are describing the situation, focus on *present,* not past, behavior, and limit the number of notations to those which are directly relevant to the present situation. You want to avoid barraging the other person with all of the remotely-related information you could offer or would like to offer. For example, you have determined that the company ends up paying your co-worker $20.00 each month for the fifteen minutes each day of non-productive time, and you know that in the past your co-worker was reprimanded for also coming in late ten minutes each day. Now, both of these facts may be true and indicative of a lack of responsibility on the other person's part, but they do not have any direct correlation to the situation at hand and what you might like to see occur as a result of your intervention. Remember, what counts is simply that you're bugged because your co-worker leaves for lunch early, you have to do all of the cleanup, and you are left without support.

The second step is to express your own feelings. That sounds contradictory to the earlier statement about avoiding concentration on the emotional consequences of negative feedback. But how *you* feel is important in clarifying how the other person's behavior is affecting you. There are two points to remember when expressing your feelings, however, that will keep this exchange from becoming an emotional battle.

The first point deals with "owning" and taking responsibility for your emotions. In the session on cognitive restructuring, it was pointed out that emotional responses develop following the occurrence of (A) an event, and (B) the internal, self-dialogue about the event, when (C) the emotional/behavioral response is created. It is the self-talk or the evaluating thoughts we have about the event that influence the way we respond either by our behavior or through our emotions. It is only fair, therefore, to take responsibility for creating them. An example of this ownership might be to say, "I feel angry and deserted when you leave early." By using "I feel" messages, the other person is not accused of causing your response and has no need to react defensively. You are simply stating how you feel.

This leads us to the second point regarding expression of emotions.

The *manner* in which feelings are relayed can be highly influential in the negative feedback process. You want to *share* how you are feeling about the event without allowing the feedback process to act as an emotional *release*. The purpose of sharing your feelings is to help the other person learn how you are responding to his behavior — not to vent your emotional energies. Having a catharsis can be fun, but it can be very dysfunctional.

Specifying the changes that you would like to see occur is the third step in the negative feedback process. Simply stating what you do not like does not guarantee that the other person will know what you want. It is appropriate to ask for a change in the other person's behavior, and the more specific you can be about this, the more likely it is to be understood by the recipient. Avoid becoming demanding, as that indicates to the recipient that she has no choice, and her response may be of a defensive or attacking nature. Simply state what you would like to have occur, such as: "I would like to request that you remain on the job until the noon hour."

The fourth and final step is to state what you perceive to be the possible consequences of a change in the other person's behavior. Tell the other person what the outcomes will be if your request is granted. For example: "If you do remain on the job until noon, I will have some assistance with the cleanup and will have some support for emergency orders. The office will run more smoothly." (See the last question in Exercise VII-1 on the next page.)

The consequences, or outcomes, are best stated in *positive* terms, avoiding "you had better do it, or else..." attitudes. Threatening the recipient with a "punishment" will not do much for consistent cooperation. It may create only a temporary compliance.

Exercise VII-1

Think of a person to whom you need to give some negative feedback. (Perhaps one of your "areas to work on" in the Assertion chapter.)

What is it exactly that you want the person to change? Describe it, so far as possible, in objective and behavioral terms.

Now, what emotion do you feel when the person behaves this way?

Next, what changes do you want? Again, describe it objectively and behaviorally.

Last, what positive consequences do you perceive as a result of the proposed change?

Use this exercise as a way to prepare to give the feedback. Your actual presentation could begin somewhat in the following way:

> " *(Name)* , I am feeling *(emotion)* about your *(current behavior)*. [Pause and give the other person a chance to respond. He may agree, and you would not have to pursue it further. If not, then . . .] I would like you to *(proposed behavior change)* . If you can do this, I think *(perceived consequences)* ."

The following is an example of a script recently followed by one of the authors:

> Amy, I am really frustrated. You keep promising that you will finish the Affirmative Action report, but I don't see it. I would appreciate it if you would set more realistic time lines and then stick to them. If you are able to do this, I won't keep after you for the reports. I'll be less tense and will stay off your back.

Another author said (in a very different situation):

> George, I am upset with your repeated propositions. Please back off a little and try a bit more courting. If you are able to do this, I may relax a bit more. I am sure we will get along better.

Now, let's look at the other side of the coin: how you can utilize this process as the recipient in a negative feedback situation. All of the concepts still apply. Your goal, as receiver of the feedback, is to objectively focus on the message being sent, in order to begin the problem-solving process.

Thus, when someone is critical of you, first use an active listening response (e.g., "you sound upset with me"). If the other responds that that indeed is the case, continue with what you perceive to be the problem. (e.g., "It sounds like you would like me to be more precise in my time lines. I think that is reasonable [or unreasonable, if that is the case].") If you need more information, ask for it. If you need help, ask. This is where your assertion training is helpful.

Exercise VII-2

Imagine that you are George (in the last example). Respond to the negative feedback given to you.

Here is another situation. You have just called your neighbor to ask for a favor, and she tells you on the phone, "Sally, I get upset with you when you always call for favors and don't return them. Please offer your services once in awhile. If you do this, I'll feel better about doing things for you. I'm sure we could be better neighbors." Respond to the negative feedback given to you.

As with earlier stress intervention techniques, the more this is practiced, the easier it becomes.

Exercise VII-3

Think of a situation where you would like to give negative feedback to another. Then:

1. Describe the situation, remembering to be specific and objective. Focus on present, not past, behaviors and only give the amount of information the recipient can use, not what you feel you have to give.

2. Express your own feelings. Focus on *sharing* this with the recipient and not as a *release* for your emotions.

3. Specify changes that you want. Try to be specific, but not demanding.

4. Share what you perceive as the consequences, or possible outcomes, of the changes that you request.

Exercise VII-4

Think of a situation where you might be the recipient of negative feedback. Then:

1. Describe the situation, remembering to be specific and objective.

2. Express your best guess of the other person's feelings.

3. Specify changes you think he might want.

4. Guess at the consequences.

Now, how would you respond?

Exercise VII-5

1. Describe how the "emotional consequences" influence a negative feedback situation.

2. Name two ways of focusing the situation toward the message to be sent.

A.

B.

3. State the four steps in the Negative Feedback process and describe how they are utilized in *giving* feedback.

A.

B.

C.

D.

4. State the four steps in the Negative Feedback process and describe how they are utilized in *receiving* feedback.

A.

B.

C.

D.

VIII

Putting It All Together

YOU HAVE NOW HAD A CHANCE to practice assessing your stressors and the resultant emotional and physiological stress, and have tried some interventions. It is our hope that you can now utilize effectively the relaxation, cognitive restructuring, active listening, and various assertive techniques. The usefulness of this stress management program is dependent on your use of these techniques in your everyday work, school, family, and/or social relationships.

In most stressful situations, you will want to employ several interventions. For instance, when someone surprises you with a sarcastic remark, you may first want to check your SUDS level and, if it is high, take a deep breath before you respond. Also, you may wish to check your self-talk. "I wonder why he said that?" is more functional than "He had no business saying that." Your first verbal response should probably be an active listening response. After the other person's response to this, an assertive statement might be the best (or you may *choose* to let the whole thing pass).

Exercise VIII-1

Return to your stress questionnaire and pick a stressor you checked as applicable for you and that you have not worked on as yet. Write it in below:

Check the interventions that you could utilize in that situation:

______ relaxation
______ cognitive restructuring
______ active listening
______ assertion
______ broken record
______ shifting gears
______ time out
______ giving negative feedback
______ receiving negative feedback

Now, here is an example of a stressor that one of the authors found difficult to deal with. (By carefully describing the situation, deciding on appropriate interventions to use, and writing a practice script, she was able to successfully manage the stress produced by the situation.)

The stressor had to do with "avoiding conflict with peers." The author's roommate was repeatedly leaving her dirty clothes all over their apartment. The faster the author picked them up, the faster her roommate deposited them. The author was able to justify not telling her roommate how she felt by saying to herself, "We're never home together for longer than thirty minutes, and I don't think it would be right to complain."

The straw that broke the camel's back, however, came one evening after the author had spent all morning cleaning and all afternoon shopping for a special dinner party. She came home with just enough time to prepare the dinner and herself before the guests arrived. The apartment was a mess: dirty clothes, dishes and newspapers deposited everywhere. And no sign of her roommate. Tomorrow would have to be the day for the author to sit down and decide what to do about it.

Here is how the situation was then described objectively and behaviorally:

> "I clean the apartment. My roommate leaves clothes and other articles about the house after using them. I end up spending more time cleaning up after her. We had agreed to share household chores equally. I end up feeling angry, frustrated and betrayed. I feel like a maid."

Using the checklist of interventions, the author decided to use relaxation techniques (her SUDS level rose to about 95 whenever she thought about it), cognitive restructuring (since she was labeling her roommate "inconsiderate"), and giving negative feedback (since she was going to tell her roommate she didn't like her behavior and wanted a change). This is how the script went:

> Taking a deep breath to bring my SUDS level down and changing my accusing thoughts to a more functional "we have a disagreement and can work it out," I will say, "Mary, I am feeling *angry* about *your leaving clothes, dishes and such about the house.* (Pause and allow Mary to respond in case she agrees with me. If not, then . . .) I would like you to *pick up and put away those things you've used before you leave the house.* If you can do this, I think *I'll feel less tense and we can have a more comfortable atmosphere at home.*"

Exercise VIII-2

Imagine you are Mary. How would you respond?

Exercise VIII-3

Pick a new situation from your "Areas to Work On" sheet. Describe the situation here as objectively and behaviorally as possible.

What is your SUDS level when this occurs?

What interventions would you use?

______ relaxation
______ cognitive restructuring
______ active listening
______ assertion
______ broken record
______ shifting gears
______ time out
______ giving negative feedback
______ receiving negative feedback

Write a script on how you propose to handle this situation in order to reduce the stress associated with it.

It is our hope that this manual has shown you effective ways to reduce negative stress in your life. As with any learning process, it will take practice and repetition to become comfortable with new ways of thinking, talking (to yourself, as well as others), and behaving. Set a realistic goal for yourself; perhaps choose a particular problem area, such as dealing with aggressive people, or learning to give and receive negative feedback, or stating your needs and wants assertively—and focus on it for a period of time, reviewing the techniques outlined in this book and repeating the accompanying exercises. When you feel comfortable with your improvements (but beware the myth of the perfect student!), move on to another area of concern. Additional copies of several of the exercises can be found at the end of this book; use them as you continue your own program of stress management.

References

I

Friedman, Meyer and Ray H. Rosenman, *Type A Behavior and Your Heart*, New York: Knopf, 1974.

Pelletier, Kenneth, *Mind as Healer, Mind as Slayer* (A Holistic Approach to Preventing Stress Disorders), New York: Delta Publishers, 1977.

II

Wolpe, J. *Psychotherapy by Reciprocal Inhibition.* Stanford: Stanford University Press, 1958.

III

Ellis, Albert and Robert A. Harper, *A Guide to Rational Living,* N. Hollywood, California: Melvin Powers, Wilshire Book Company, 1975.

Ellis, Albert, *Reason and Emotion in Psychotherapy,* Seacaucus, New Jersey: Lyle Stuart, Inc. 1975.

Goodman, David S., and Maxie E. Maulsby, Jr., *Emotional Well-Being Rational Behavior Training,* Springfield, Illinois: Charles C. Thomas, 1974.

IV

Rogers, C.R., *Client-Centered Therapy,* Bostón: Houghton Mifflin, 1951.

V

Lange, A., and Jakubowski, P., *Responsible Assertive Behavior,* Champaign, Ill.: Research Press, 1976.

Wolpe, J., *The Practice of Behavior Therapy,* New York: Pergamon Press, 1973.

Appendix

CONFLICT/STRESS QUESTIONNAIRE

I. STRESS SYMPTOMS

Which of these stress symptoms do you experience? Circle the appropriate number. The column after the "5" indicates whether it represents P (physiological stress), E (emotional stress), or B (behavioral stress).

	NEVER	RARELY	SOMETIMES	OFTEN	ALWAYS	
Headaches	1	2	3	4	5	(P)
Stomach aches or tension	1	2	3	4	5	(P)
Backaches	1	2	3	4	5	(P)
Stiffness in the neck and shoulders	1	2	3	4	5	(P)
Elevated blood pressure	1	2	3	4	5	(P)
Fatigue	1	2	3	4	5	(P)
Crying	1	2	3	4	5	(B)
Forgetfulness	1	2	3	4	5	(B)
Yelling	1	2	3	4	5	(B)
Blaming	1	2	3	4	5	(B)
Bossiness	1	2	3	4	5	(B)
Compulsive gum chewing	1	2	3	4	5	(B)
Compulsive eating	1	2	3	4	5	(B)
Worrying	1	2	3	4	5	(E)
Depression	1	2	3	4	5	(E)
Agitation	1	2	3	4	5	(B)
Impatience	1	2	3	4	5	(E)
Anger	1	2	3	4	5	(B)
Frustration	1	2	3	4	5	(E)
Loneliness	1	2	3	4	5	(E)
Powerlessness	1	2	3	4	5	(E)
Inflexibility	1	2	3	4	5	(E)
Compulsive smoking	1	2	3	4	5	(B)
Teeth grinding	1	2	3	4	5	(B)
Other ________________	1	2	3	4	5	

II. STRESS REDUCTION

How often do you use these measures to relax?

	NEVER	RARELY	SOMETIMES	OFTEN	ALWAYS
Take aspirin	1	2	3	4	5
Use tranquilizers or other medication	1	2	3	4	5
Drink coffee, Coke, or eat frequently	1	2	3	4	5
Use relaxation techniques (meditation, yoga)	1	2	3	4	5
Use informal relaxation techniques (e.g., take time out for deep breathing, imagining pleasant scenes)	1	2	3	4	5

	NEVER	RARELY	SOMETIMES	OFTEN	ALWAYS
Exercise	1	2	3	4	5
Talk to someone you know	1	2	3	4	5
Leave your work area and go somewhere (time out, sick days, lunch away from your organization, etc.)	1	2	3	4	5

	NEVER	RARELY	SOMETIMES	OFTEN	ALWAYS
Smoke	1	2	3	4	5
Use humor	1	2	3	4	5
Have an alcoholic drink	1	2	3	4	5
Other ________________	1	2	3	4	5

III. STRESSFUL CONDITIONS

There are frequently day to day conditions which we find stressful. Go through them, reading each one, and put a check next to those that apply to you. Then go back over the checked items and indicate how often each source is true for you by circling the appropriate number.

The symbols in parentheses indicate the type of stressors: *P* (physical), *S* (social), *O* (organizational), and *ST* (self-talk).

	NEVER	RARELY	SOMETIMES	OFTEN	ALWAYS
____ 1. I am uncomfortable meeting strangers (S)/(ST)	1	2	3	4	5
____ 2. I am uncomfortable speaking in front of a group (ST)	1	2	3	4	5
____ 3. I am concerned over my ability to do everything I want to (ST)	1	2	3	4	5
____ 4. Others I work with seem unclear about what my job is (O)	1	2	3	4	5
____ 5. I have differences of opinions with my supervisors (O)/(S)	1	2	3	4	5
____ 6. Others' demands for my time at work are in conflict with each other (O)	1	2	3	4	5
____ 7. I lack confidence in "management" (O)	1	2	3	4	5
____ 8. "Management" expects me to interrupt my work for new priorities (O)	1	2	3	4	5
____ 9. There is conflict between my unit and others I must work with (O)	1	2	3	4	5
____10. I only get feedback when my performance is unsatisfactory (S)	1	2	3	4	5
____11. Decisions or changes which affect me are made "above" without my knowledge or involvement (O)	1	2	3	4	5
____12. I have too much to do and too little time to do it (ST)	1	2	3	4	5
____13. I feel overqualified for the work I actually do (ST)	1	2	3	4	5
____14. I feel underqualified for the work I actually do (ST)	1	2	3	4	5

	NEVER	RARELY	SOMETIMES	OFTEN	ALWAYS
____15. The people I work with closely are trained in a different field than mine (O)	1	2	3	4	5
____16. I must go to other departments to get my job done (O)	1	2	3	4	5
____17. I have unsettled conflicts with people in my department (or family) (S)	1	2	3	4	5
____18. I have unsettled conflicts with other departments (O)/(S)	1	2	3	4	5
____19. I get little personal support from the people I work with (S)	1	2	3	4	5
____20. I spend my time "fighting fires" rather than working to a plan (O)	1	2	3	4	5
____21. I feel family pressure about long hours, weekend work, etc. (S)	1	2	3	4	5
____22. I have self-imposed demands to meet scheduled deadlines (ST)	1	2	3	4	5
____23. I have difficulty giving negative feedback to peers (S)	1	2	3	4	5
____24. I have difficulty giving negative feedback to subordinates (or children) (S)	1	2	3	4	5
____25. I have difficulty dealing with agressive people (S)	1	2	3	4	5
____26. I have difficulty dealing with passive people (S)	1	2	3	4	5
____27. Overlapping responsibilities cause me problems (O)	1	2	3	4	5
____28. I am uncomfortable arbitrating a conflict among my peers (S)	1	2	3	4	5
____29. I am uncomfortable arbitrating a conflict among my subordinates (or children) (S)	1	2	3	4	5
____30. I avoid conflicts with peers (S)	1	2	3	4	5
____31. I avoid conflicts with superiors (S)	1	2	3	4	5
____32. I avoid conflicts with subordinates (S)	1	2	3	4	5
____33. Allocation of resources generates conflict in my organization (O)	1	2	3	4	5
____34. I experience frustration with conflicting procedures (O)	1	2	3	4	5
____35. My personal needs are in conflict with the organization (O)/(ST)	1	2	3	4	5
____36. I am bothered by my noisy environment (P)	1	2	3	4	5
____37. I have difficulty staying focused on a task (ST)	1	2	3	4	5
____38. My wife (husband) makes too many demands on me (S)	1	2	3	4	5
____39. I have concern over my parents' health (S)	1	2	3	4	5
____40. I have difficulty communicating with my children (S)	1	2	3	4	5
____41. I have difficulty saying what I feel (ST)	1	2	3	4	5

M-K Assertive-Aggressive Inventory

The M-K Assertive-Aggressive Inventory is designed to provide information to an individual regarding the way he/she relates on the job to bosses, coworkers and subordinates. The behaviors identified are assertive, aggressive, or non-assertive.

For each statement, the individual is asked to rank on a scale of 0-4 how he/she responds in a given situation.

Assertive Behavior—By assertive behavior we mean the ability to express one's feelings, to choose how one will act, speak up for his/her rights in an appropriate, non-defensive way.

Aggressive behavior—By aggressive behavior we mean that it aims at hurting another person, physically or emotionally, and results in one winner at the expense of another's self-esteem.

Non-assertive behavior—By non-assertive behavior we mean passive behavior such as when one retreats from a situation, avoids conflict and blames others for what is happening.

Positive features: One of the outstanding features of the instrument is that it points out an individual's way of behaving towards three distinct groups: bosses, coworkers and subordinates. It is fairly simple to score.

On the last page is a score sheet for recording the scores from the left hand side of the M-K Inventory.

Marcia Manter
Rose Kennedy

Rating Instructions

Please answer the questions by rating each statement on a scale of 0 to 4. Place your rankings on the left side of the appropriate statement.

Remember, your answer should reflect how you generally express yourself in a variety of situations.

If a particular situation does not apply to you, answer as you think you would respond in that situation. Your answer should *not* reflect how you feel you "ought to act" or how you would "like to act."

Do not deliberate over any individual statement. Please work quickly. Your first response to the statement is probably your most accurate one. Most people finish in about fifteen minutes.

RATING SCALE

Almost Always or Always	*Usually*	*Sometimes*	*Seldom*	*Never or Rarely*
(4)	(3)	(2)	(1)	(0)

____ 1. I complain to others about the ineptness of my boss.

____ 2. If a subordinate makes a statement that I consider untrue, I question him/her out loud.

____ 3. I feel good after I vent my anger when I tell off a subordinate when he/she really messes up a simple job.

____ 4. I am quick to tell a coworker whenever he/she has done something that makes my job easier.

____ 5. If my boss ignores a request, I ask until I get an answer.

____ 6. When a subordinate does something on the job that I don't like, I resort to name calling.

____ 7. I feel free to initiate a discussion with my boss about my performance on the job.

____ 8. I find it difficult to ask a subordinate to do a favor for me.

RATING SCALE

Almost Always or Always	*Usually*	*Sometimes*	*Seldom*	*Never or Rarely*
(4)	(3)	(2)	(1)	(0)

____ 9. I complain to others about the ineptness of subordinates.

____ 10. I find it difficult to ask a coworker to do a favor for me.

____ 11. I have trouble asking for time off, even if it is justified.

____ 12. I find myself grumbling about my boss' behavior.

____ 13. If a coworker makes a remark that I don't really understand but think might be an insult, I question him/her about the meaning.

____ 14. I have trouble thinking of what to say when my boss compliments me on a good job.

____ 15. I tell my boss when he/she does something on the job that in my judgement is an error.

____ 16. I make fun of subordinates to others.

____ 17. If a coworker ignores a request, I ask again until I get an answer.

____ 18. I feel good after I vent my anger by telling off the boss when he/she really messes up a simple situation.

____ 19. I tell subordinates when they do something on the job that is an error in my judgement.

____ 20. When something goes wrong on the job, I am quick to blame the boss.

____ 21. If a group of subordinates confronts me on an issue, I stand firm on my position.

____ 22. I become nervous when I talk to my boss about a problem.

____ 23. I make fun of my coworkers to others.

____ 24. When my boss does something on the job that I don't like, I resort to name calling.

RATING SCALE

Almost Always or Always	*Usually*	*Sometimes*	*Seldom*	*Never or Rarely*
(4)	(3)	(2)	(1)	(0)

____ 25. I find myself grumbling about my coworkers' behavior.

____ 26. I feel free to initiate a discussion with subordinates about their performance on the job.

____ 27. I have difficulty saying no when a coworker makes what I consider to be an unreasonable request.

____ 28. I find it difficult to ask my boss to do a favor for me.

____ 29. If a coworker makes a statement that I consider to be untrue, I question him/her out loud.

____ 30. When something goes wrong on the job, I am quick to blame a subordinate.

____ 31. I make fun of my boss to others.

____ 32. I avoid speaking up when a subordinate has done something that makes my job harder.

____ 33. If my boss makes a statement that I consider untrue, I question him/her out loud.

____ 34. If a subordinate ignores a request, I ask again until I get an answer.

____ 35. When something goes wrong on the job, I am quick to blame a coworker.

____ 36. I find myself shouting at a subordinate.

____ 37. I tell a coworker when he/she has done something on the job that in my judgement is an error.

____ 38. If a subordinate makes a remark that I don't really understand but think might be an insult, I question her/him about the meaning.

____ 39. I complain to others about the ineptness of coworkers.

RATING SCALE

Almost Always or Always	*Usually*	*Sometimes*	*Seldom*	*Never or Rarely*
(4)	(3)	(2)	(1)	(0)

____ 40. I have difficulty saying no when a subordinate makes what I consider an unreasonable request.

____ 41. I become nervous when I talk to a subordinate about a problem.

____ 42. If a boss makes a remark to me that I don't really understand but I think might be an insult, I question her/him about the meaning.

____ 43. I feel free to initiate a discussion with coworkers about their performance on a joint program.

____ 44. I grant subordinates requests for time off, even when it is not justified.

____ 45. I avoid saying something when a coworker has done something that makes my job harder.

____ 46. I find myself shouting at a coworker.

____ 47. I avoid saying something when my boss has done something that makes my job harder.

____ 48. I have trouble thinking of what to say when a coworker compliments me on a good job.

____ 49. I have difficulty saying no when my boss makes what I consider an unreasonable request.

____ 50. I am quick to tell my boss whenever he/she has done something that makes my job easier.

____ 51. I feel good after I vent my anger by telling off a coworker when he/she really messes up a simple job.

____ 52. I become nervous when I talk to a coworker about a problem.

RATING SCALE

Almost Always or Always	*Usually*	*Sometimes*	*Seldom*	*Never or Rarely*
(4)	(3)	(2)	(1)	(0)

____ 53. When a coworker does something on the job that I don't like, I resort to name calling.

____ 54. When coworkers confront me regarding my performance, I refuse to listen.

M-K Assertive-Aggressive Inventory

SCORE SHEET

	Assertive Behavior		*Non-Assertive Behavior*		*Aggressive Behavior*	
	5.	______	11.	______	1.	______
	7.	______	14.	______	12.	______
Towards the Boss	15.	______	22.	______	18.	______
	33.	______	28.	______	20.	______
	42.	______	47.	______	24.	______
	50.	______	49.	______	31.	______
	TOTAL	______	TOTAL	______	TOTAL	______
	13.	______	10.	______	23.	______
	17.	______	27.	______	35.	______
Towards one's Coworkers	19.	______	45.	______	39.	______
	29.	______	48.	______	46.	______
	37.	______	52.	______	51.	______
	43.	______	54.	______	53.	______
	TOTAL	______	TOTAL	______	TOTAL	______

	2. ________	8. ________	3. ________
	4. ________	25. ________	6. ________
Towards one's Subordinates	21. ________	32. ________	9. ________
	26. ________	40. ________	16. ________
	34. ________	41. ________	30. ________
	38. ________	44. ________	36. ________
	TOTAL ______	TOTAL ______	TOTAL ______

16-24 HIGH
8-16 MODERATE
1-8 LOW

Think of the last time you were feeling a strong, unpleasant emotion. Write that emotion under C in the following diagram. Now, under A, write in the event that happened before the emotion occurred. Finally, under B, put your best guess as to what you were thinking between the event and the emotion. Was your thinking rational? Was it functional, i.e., did it help you?

A — ACTIVATING EVENT

B — YOUR THINKING

C — FEELINGS AND BEHAVIOR

Review the criteria that distinguishes between rational and irrational thinking and continue.

D — OBJECTIVE EVENT

E — YOUR RATIONAL THINKING

F — YOUR DESIRED FEELINGS AND BEHAVIOR

Think of the last time you were feeling a strong, unpleasant emotion. Write that emotion under C in the following diagram. Now, under A, write in the event that happened before the emotion occurred. Finally, under B, put your best guess as to what you were thinking between the event and the emotion. Was your thinking rational? Was it functional, i.e., did it help you?

A — ACTIVATING EVENT

____

____

____

↓

B — YOUR THINKING

____

____

____

↓

C — FEELINGS AND BEHAVIOR

____

____

____

Review the criteria that distinguishes between rational and irrational thinking and continue.

D — OBJECTIVE EVENT

____

____

____

↓

E — YOUR RATIONAL THINKING

____

____

____

↓

F — YOUR DESIRED FEELINGS AND BEHAVIOR

____

____

____

EXERCISE III-2

(a) List your major roles, in descending order of their importance to you.

ROLES

1. ______________________________
2. ______________________________
3. ______________________________
4. ______________________________
5. ______________________________
6. ______________________________

(b) Now, with respect to each of the first three, the ones you assigned highest priority, list *your* major role myths.

1. ROLE NO. 1 ______________________

MAJOR MYTHS

a. ______________________________
b. ______________________________
c. ______________________________
d. ______________________________
e. ______________________________

2. ROLE NO. 2 ______________________

MAJOR MYTHS

a. ______________________________
b. ______________________________
c. ______________________________
d. ______________________________
e. ______________________________

3. ROLE NO. 3 ____________________

MAJOR MYTHS

a. ____________________

b. ____________________

c. ____________________

d. ____________________

e. ____________________

EXERCISE III-2

(a) List your major roles, in descending order of their importance to you.

ROLES

1. ____________________
2. ____________________
3. ____________________
4. ____________________
5. ____________________
6. ____________________

(b) Now, with respect to each of the first three, the ones you assigned highest priority, list *your* major role myths.

1. ROLE NO. 1 ____________________

MAJOR MYTHS

a. ____________________

b. ____________________

c. ____________________

d. ____________________

e. ____________________

2. ROLE NO. 2 ____________________

MAJOR MYTHS

a. ____________________

b. ____________________

c. ____________________

d. ____________________

e. ____________________

3. ROLE NO. 3 ______________________________

MAJOR MYTHS

a. ______________________________

b. ______________________________

c. ______________________________

d. ______________________________

e. ______________________________

EXERCISE III-5

Return to the irrational beliefs that you circled earlier. Write down one of them.

Belief:

Write down as many reasons as you can why this belief is irrational.

Challenge:

Now, rewrite the belief to one which is more reasonable.

New Belief:

Pick one more for practice.

Belief:

Challenge:

New Belief:

EXERCISE III-5

Return to the irrational beliefs that you circled earlier. Write down one of them.

Belief:

Write down as many reasons as you can why this belief is irrational.

Challenge:

Now, rewrite the belief to one which is more reasonable.

New Belief:

Pick one more for practice.

Belief:

Challenge:

New Belief:

EXERCISE V-4

(1) Write a short script on a situation which causes your SUDS level to go to 75 or above. (2) Try some problem-solving and ask yourself whether an assertive behavior response would help relieve your anxiety. (3) Write down what that response would be.

SITUATION:

ASSERTIVE RESPONSE:

EXERCISE V-4

(1) Write a short script on a situation which causes your SUDS level to go to 75 or above. (2) Try some problem-solving and ask yourself whether an assertive behavior response would help relieve your anxiety. (3) Write down what that response would be.

SITUATION:

ASSERTIVE RESPONSE:

EXERCISE VII-1

Think of a person to whom you need to give some negative feedback. (Perhaps one of your "areas to work on" in the assertion chapter.)

What is it exactly that you want the person to change? Describe it, so far as possible, in objective and behavioral terms.

Now, what emotion do you feel when the person behaves this way?

Next, what changes do you want? Again, describe it objectively and behaviorally.

Last, what positive consequences do you perceive as a result of the proposed change?

EXERCISE VII-1

Think of a person to whom you need to give some negative feedback. (Perhaps one of your "areas to work on" in the assertion chapter.)

What is it exactly that you want the person to change? Describe it, so far as possible, in objective and behavioral terms.

Now, what emotion do you feel when the person behaves this way?

Next, what changes do you want? Again, describe it objectively and behaviorally.

Last, what positive consequences do you perceive as a result of the proposed change?

EXERCISE VII-3

Think of a situation where you would like to give negative feedback to another. Then:

1. Describe the situation, remembering to be specific and objective. Focus on present, not past, behaviors and only give the amount of information the recipient can use, not what you feel you have to give.

2. Express your own feelings. Focus on *sharing* this with the recipient and not as a *release* for your emotions.

3. Specify changes that you want. Try to be specific, but not demanding.

4. Share what you perceive as the consequences, or possible outcomes, of the changes that you request.

EXERCISE VII-3

Think of a situation where you would like to give negative feedback to another. Then:

1. Describe the situation, remembering to be specific and objective. Focus on present, not past, behaviors and only give the amount of information the recipient can use, not what you feel you have to give.

2. Express your own feelings. Focus on *sharing* this with the recipient and not as a *release* for your emotions.

3. Specify changes that you want. Try to be specific, but not demanding.

4. Share what you perceive as the consequences, or possible outcomes, of the changes that you request.

Use this exercise as a way to prepare to give negative feedback.

______________________, I am feeling ______________________

about your ______________________

I would like you to ______________________

If you can do this, I think ______________________

____

______________________, I am feeling ______________________

about your ______________________

I would like you to ______________________

If you can do this, I think ______________________

____

______________________, I am feeling ______________________

about your ______________________

I would like you to ______________________

If you can do this, I think ______________________

____

______________________, I am feeling ______________________

about your ______________________

I would like you to ______________________

If you can do this, I think ______________________

____

EXERCISE VII-4

Think of a situation where you might be the recipient of negative feedback. Then:

1. Describe the situation, remembering to be specific and objective.

2. Express your best guess of the other person's feelings.

3. Specify changes you think he might want.

4. Guess at the consequences.

Now, how would you respond?

EXERCISE VII-4

Think of a situation where you might be the recipient of negative feedback. Then:

1. Describe the situation, remembering to be specific and objective.

2. Express your best guess of the other person's feelings.

3. Specify changes you think he might want.

4. Guess at the consequences.

Now, how would you respond?

EXERCISE VIII-3

Pick a new situation from your "Areas to Work On" sheet. Describe the situation here as objectively and behaviorally as possible.

What is your SUDS level when this occurs?

What interventions would you use?

______relaxation
______cognitive restructuring
______active listening
______assertion
______broken record
______shifting gears
______time out
______giving negative feedback
______receiving negative feedback

Write a script on how you propose to handle this situation in order to reduce the stress associated with it.

EXERCISE VIII-3

Pick a new situation from your "Areas to Work On" sheet. Describe the situation here as objectively and behaviorally as possible.

What is your SUDS level when this occurs?

What interventions would you use?

_______relaxation
_______cognitive restructuring
_______active listening
_______assertion
_______broken record
_______shifting gears
_______time out
_______giving negative feedback
_______receiving negative feedback

Write a script on how you propose to handle this situation in order to reduce the stress associated with it.

AREAS TO WORK ON

Situation	People Involved	Typical Behavior Response	Desired Behavior	Present SUDS Level

AREAS TO WORK ON

Situation	People Involved	Typical Behavior Response	Desired Behavior	Present SUDS Level